Springer Series on Child and Family Studies

Series Editor

Nirbhay N. Singh, Medical College of Georgia
Augusta University
Augusta, GA, USA

The Springer Series on Child and Family Studies addresses fundamental psychological, educational, social, and related issues within the context of child and family research. Volumes published in this series examine clinical topics with an additional focus on epidemiological, developmental, and life span issues. Leading scholars explore such factors as race and immigration, parenting, and the effects of war and violence on military families and unite a vast literature into a comprehensive series of related research volumes.

Bridget A. Makol • Junhui Yang
Mo Wang • Andres De Los Reyes

Youth Development in Context

Integrating Multiple Informants to Assess Behavior

Springer

Bridget A. Makol
Department of Pediatrics
Rush University Medical Center
Chicago, IL, USA

Junhui Yang
Warrington College of Business
University of Florida
Gainesville, FL, USA

Mo Wang
Warrington College of Business
University of Florida
Gainesville, FL, USA

Andres De Los Reyes
Department of Psychology
University of Maryland, College Park
College Park, MD, USA

ISSN 2570-0421 ISSN 2570-043X (electronic)
Springer Series on Child and Family Studies
ISBN 978-3-031-80548-6 ISBN 978-3-031-80549-3 (eBook)
https://doi.org/10.1007/978-3-031-80549-3

This Springer imprint is published by the registered company Springer Nature Switzerland AG
The registered company address is: Gewerbestrasse 11, 6330 Cham, Switzerland

About the Book

This book probes the most common approach to assessing behavior in youth development. It explores use of multiple informants who each observe youth in the social contexts that typify their everyday lives, including parents, teachers, peers, and youth themselves. The book characterizes the most common outcome from taking this assessment approach—the discrepant results or estimates about behavior that informants' reports often produce—and describes the distinct strategies researchers have historically used to integrate these data. This conceptually grounded, thoroughly resourced, and methodologically rigorous book provides readers with a paradigm for testing competing data integration strategies, using a sophisticated suite of Monte Carlo simulation and measurement validation tools that are applicable to a host of assessment scenarios in scholarship on youth development.

Key areas of coverage include:

- Use of multiple informants to assess behavior in youth development
- The frequent observation of discrepant results when assessing behavior in youth development
- Theoretical models for explaining discrepant results in behavioral assessments
- How theoretical models inform strategies for integrating assessment data
- Key distinctions in the assumptions that underlie the use of competing integrative strategies
- Application of Monte Carlo simulation strategies for testing competing integrative strategies
- Application of measurement validation procedures for testing competing integrative strategies
- Key directions for future research on assessing behavior in youth development

This book is an essential resource for researchers, professors, graduate students as well as clinicians, therapists, and other professionals in developmental psychology, social work, public health, pediatrics, family studies, child and adolescent psychiatry, school and educational psychology, and all interrelated disciplines.

Contents

About the Authors

Bridget A. Makol received her Ph.D. from the University of Maryland and is Assistant Professor of Pediatrics and Psychology at Rush University Medical Center. Her research interests revolve around assessing youth mental health, with an emphasis on depression and anxiety.

Junhui Yang is a doctoral student in the Department of Management at the University of Florida. Her research interests revolve around advanced quantitative methodologies and their applications to applied problems, with an emphasis on personnel selection in workplace settings.

Mo Wang received his Ph.D. from Bowling Green State University and is University Distinguished Professor of Management at the University of Florida. His research addresses issues surrounding retirement and older worker employment, occupational health psychology, expatriate and newcomer adjustment, leadership and team processes, and advanced quantitative methodologies.

Andres De Los Reyes received his Ph.D. from Yale University and is Professor of Psychology at the University of Maryland, where he serves as Director of the Comprehensive Assessment and Intervention Program. His research focuses on understanding the discrepant results that mental health assessments commonly produce. He is a Fulbright Scholar, two-term Editor-in-Chief of the *Journal of Clinical Child and Adolescent Psychology* (2017–2026), Co-Chair (with Ye Tong) of the Sixth Edition of *The Standards for Educational and Psychological Testing*, and the author of the 2024 books *Discrepant Results in Mental Health Research* (Oxford University Press) and *The Early Career Researcher's Toolbox* (Springer).

Chapter 1
Use of Multiple Informants to Assess Behavior in Youth Development

Assessing child and adolescent (i.e., youth) behavior is a complex task. The behavioral domains of interest to scholars in youth development—psychosocial strengths, family environments, peer relations, academic achievement, and mental health, for example—require understanding behaviors within the social contexts in which they manifest (see Achenbach et al., 1987; Gresham et al., 2010; Hawker & Boulton, 2000; Hou et al., 2020; Ivanova et al., 2022; Talbott et al., 2023). Youth vary not only in the contexts that encompass their social worlds, but also in how or why they react as they do. Thus, understanding youth behavior requires consideration of various facets of development, all within the social contexts that youth navigate day to day. The complexity underlying youth behavior highlights the need for precise and psychometrically sound assessment tools (De Los Reyes et al., 2017, 2023a; De Los Reyes & Makol, 2022; Hunsley & Mash, 2007).

Given the complexity of youth behavior, there exists no single tool to index it (e.g., Achenbach, 2020; De Los Reyes, 2011; Kagan et al., 2002; Richters, 1992). Consequently, accurately characterizing youth behavior in context-sensitive ways requires multi-dimensional and multi-method approaches to assessment. In both research and applied settings, the most widely used, context-sensitive approach entails soliciting reports from multiple informants (e.g., parents, teachers, youth, peers). These informants observe youth in unique contexts (e.g., home, school, peer interactions; Achenbach et al., 1987). As such, their use as valid data sources hinges on the degree to which each informant contributes incrementally valid information about the youth undergoing evaluation (Hunsley & Mash, 2007). The uniqueness of each report invariably results in a key task—that of integrating reports (Wright et al., 2022). This task informs decision-making across research and applied settings. This book represents the most conceptually grounded, methodologically rigorous, and authoritative test to date of the validity of widely used strategies for integrating data from assessments of youth behavior.

B. A. Makol et al., *Youth Development in Context*, Springer Series on Child and Family Studies, https://doi.org/10.1007/978-3-031-80549-3_1

1.1 Discrepant Results and the Data Conditions That Typify Assessments of Youth Behavior

Data from multi-informant reports serve foundational roles in both basic and applied research in youth development. In basic research, researchers use these reports to index a variety of domains (e.g., mental health, parenting, social skills, peer relations) and to address many research aims relevant to youth development, including the causes, consequences, and predictors of developmental outcomes and their etiologies (e.g., De Los Reyes et al., 2019a; Korelitz & Garber, 2016; Renk & Phares, 2004; Rescorla et al., 2013; Watts et al., 2022). In applied research, scholars rely on multi-informant reports to inform decision-making scenarios of various kinds, including diagnosis and classification of youth mental health, identification of evidence-based interventions, and delivery of educational programming (e.g., Talbott et al., 2023; Weisz et al., 2005; Youngstrom & Van Meter, 2016).

Across basic and applied research scenarios, scholars must contend with perhaps the most robust outcome resulting from the use of multi-informant data. Decades of work reveal that multi-informant reports commonly yield unique estimates of youth behavior (i.e., *discrepant results*; De Los Reyes, 2024). By "unique estimates," we mean that informants often differ in the quantitative estimates they provide about the same domain. For instance, a parent rates their child's hyperactivity as "10" on a ten-point scale, whereas the child's teacher rates their hyperactivity as "4" on that same scale. These differences in estimates often translate into distinct impressions and decisions about behavior. For instance, symptom endorsements for a youth's anxiety based on youth self-report may lead to a diagnosis, but independent assessments based on the endorsements of their parent may not (see also De Los Reyes & Kazdin, 2005). Discrepant results in qualitative judgments traverse a host of decision-making scenarios. That is, researchers often arrive at distinct conclusions about risk and protective factors for youth mental health concerns, evidence-based interventions to address these concerns, and decisions surrounding treatment planning (for reviews, see De Los Reyes & Kazdin, 2006, 2008; De Los Reyes & Makol, 2022; De Los Reyes et al., 2022a). In education, researchers encounter discrepant results on a host of indices relevant to placement in educational programs and determining successful academic outcomes (see also Talbott et al., 2023).

As an example of the robust nature of discrepant results, consider assessments of youth mental health. Meta-analyses of multi-informant reports of youth mental health consistently reveal low-to-moderate levels of convergence (i.e., *r*s = .20 s–.30 s; Achenbach et al., 1987; De Los Reyes et al., 2015, 2013a). Meta-analyses also reveal that these discrepancies appear across behavioral domains, not just mental health domains. Multi-informant assessments produce discrepant results, regardless of the developmental period of those assessed, the domain assessed, informants used, measures used, and where in the world the assessment occurred (e.g., Achenbach et al., 2005; De Los Reyes et al., 2019b; Hendriks et al., 2018; Hou et al., 2020; Korelitz & Garber, 2016; Renk & Phares, 2004; Rescorla et al., 2013, 2017; Romano et al., 2018; Stratis & Lecavalier, 2015; Sudkamp et al.,

2012). No decision-making setting (e.g., laboratory, legislative office, hospital, community mental health center, parent-teacher conference) is immune from encountering discrepant results.

When interpreting the discrepant results produced by assessments of youth behavior, it is important to consider that they occur within a set of *data conditions*. By "data conditions," we mean characteristics of multi-informant reports that set the foundations for how to understand and interpret the results produced by behavioral assessments. These characteristics reveal that discrepant results are not vestiges of how scholars have historically assessed youth behavior. Discrepant results are here to stay. Discrepant results are not unique to multi-informant data (see De Los Reyes, 2024; De Los Reyes & Aldao, 2015; De Los Reyes et al., 2020; Clarkson et al., 2020; Kaurin et al., 2022; Meyer et al., 2001; Talbott et al., 2023). Further, prior work indicates that discrepant results are often byproducts of sound and comprehensive assessment processes.

Consider that the level of discrepant results has remained stable over the course of several decades (cf. Achenbach et al., 1987; De Los Reyes et al., 2015). We know that the stability of discrepant results is unlikely explained by issues with faulty instrumentation, because the number of well-established instruments to assess youth behavior has increased, not decreased, over these decades (De Los Reyes, Epkins, et al., 2023b). Relatedly, current meta-analytic reviews of discrepant results involve estimating these discrepancies from studies using assessments that not only contain well-established or thoroughly vetted instruments, but also informants who provide psychometrically sound reports (see also Achenbach, 2020). Further, youth navigate many social contexts in their day-to-day lives, not just one. Assessing youth behavior while also considering these contexts requires reports from informants who vary from each other in where they observe youth (e.g., home, school, peer interactions). Quantitative methodologists refer to these data sources as *structurally different informants* (Eid et al., 2008). By construction, what makes these informants structurally differ from each other must be pertinent or relevant to the assessment task—to understand the domains that characterize youth behavior (e.g., social skills, family conflict, peer victimization, school grades, anxiety). These data conditions reveal the logic behind contemporary approaches to assessing youth behavior and interpreting the discrepant results produced by these assessments. When informants provide context-sensitive, unique, and psychometrically sound reports about youth, the discrepancies between their reports likely contain valid data about youth behavior. That is, discrepant results may contain *domain-relevant information* (for a review, see De Los Reyes et al., 2023a).

The data conditions that typify multi-informant assessments of youth behavior reveal a key bottleneck in scholarship in youth development. No empirically based consensus guidelines exist for interpreting discrepant results and, importantly, using the data they contain to optimize the accuracy of decision-making (Phares & Hankinson, 2020; Talbott et al., 2023). In fact, underlying this lack of guidelines is a series of tensions in the literature, namely, among (a) researchers' theories about what discrepant results reflect, (b) the evidence supporting these theories, and (c) the strategies used to integrate multi-informant data.

1.2 Rater Bias Models and the Usage Assumptions of Integrative Strategies

Historically, the theoretical models most often used to study discrepant results and guide the integration of multi-informant data are what we refer to in this book as *rater bias models*. That is, any systematic differences that exist between informants' reports (e.g., parent report > teacher report on ratings of a child's hyperactivity) reflect factors that do not accurately reflect the domains that informants rate. Let us return to the parent-teacher discrepancies in reports about a child's hyperactivity. One could interpret these differences as potentially arising from true differences in the child's behavior in different social contexts (i.e., parent at home vs. teacher at school). Yet, rater bias models hold that these differences reflect factors that are irrelevant to understanding the child's behavior (for a review, see De Los Reyes et al., 2022b). As such, rater bias models approach discrepant results as "nuisance variance" that must be eliminated, reduced, or otherwise accounted for when integrating data from multiple informants or sources.

In youth development, the most frequently cited rater bias model is the *depression→distortion hypothesis* (Richters, 1992)—the notion that when an informant's mental state is typified by low mood or increased stress, this negatively impacts their ability to accurately observe behavior, encode it in memory, and retrieve it from memory to provide reports. Further, the model posits that such a state will lead to an informant making more negative reports about youth behavior (e.g., increased youth anxiety, decreased youth social skills, increased negative parenting), relative to other informants who are not depressed or undergoing high stress. For decades, the depression→distortion hypothesis has guided researchers in work on discrepant results, including work across periods of youth development (e.g., Berg-Nielsen et al., 2003, 2012; Booth et al., 2023; Boyle & Pickles, 1997; Briggs-Gowan et al., 1996; Castagna et al., 2020; Chi & Hinshaw, 2002; Chilcoat & Breslau, 1997; De Los Reyes et al., 2008; De Los Reyes & Prinstein, 2004; Durbin & Wilson, 2012; Gartstein et al., 2009; Kroes et al., 2003; Madsen et al., 2020; Najman et al., 2000; Olino et al., 2020, 2021; Treutler & Epkins, 2003; Wesselhoeft et al., 2021; Youngstrom et al., 1999). In fact, rater bias models like the depression→distortion hypothesis have been so influential to scholarship in youth development that they have compelled scholars to develop analytic modeling procedures that they claim "correct" for discrepant results (see Müller & Furniss, 2013; Müller et al., 2014).

Being the most widely studied rater bias model, it is important to note three things about the depression→distortion hypothesis. First, it rests on a meager foundation of empirical support. That is, studies guided by the depression→distortion hypothesis either find mixed support for the hypothesis or null findings, particularly when scholars have used experimental or laboratory-controlled approaches to testing the hypothesis (for a review, see De Los Reyes & Makol, 2022). As an example, consider that among the most well-conducted studies that have tested the depression→distortion hypothesis, even the authors of this study contended that the magnitudes of rater distortions they observed would not be compelling enough to decline to use an informant that is deemed to provide "distorted" ratings of youth behavior (Youngstrom et al., 1999).

Second, part of the reason why empirical support for the depression→distortion hypothesis is as weak as it is stems from a key limitation of the hypothesis itself. The depression→distortion hypothesis does not address the notion that the informants who make reports about youth are often significant others in their lives (e.g., parents, teachers). Several decades of studies in youth development very clearly indicate that the functioning of significant others impacts how youth behave (Atkins et al., 2017; Carlone & Milan, 2021; Cicchetti, 1984; Goodman et al., 2020; Luthar et al., 2000). As such, findings that appear to support the depression→distortion hypothesis may be parsimoniously interpreted as reflecting a key reality about youth: How youth function may depend, in part, on how others in their lives function.

Third, the hypothesis' key premise—that all discrepant results reflect rater biases—is violated by not only the data conditions that typify assessments of youth behavior, but also the lack of a "gold standard" or even psychometrically sound ways to detect rater biases (see Richters, 1992). Without the ability to accurately detect rater biases, researchers guided by the depression→distortion hypothesis are left to assume that if they detect a relation between an informant's mood and discrepant results, then the relation reflects rater biases and nothing more. Importantly, this would be an assumption that researchers cannot test in any empirically sound way. In this respect, the interpretation of these effects lacks the ability to be falsified (see also Haeffel et al., 2022). If an interpretation cannot be falsified, then a scholar guided by the depression→distortion hypothesis may mischaracterize discrepant results as reflecting useless data when these discrepancies, in fact, contain useful or domain-relevant data (see also De Los Reyes, 2024; De Los Reyes et al., 2023a).

Taken together, several factors make it unlikely that rater bias models accurately characterize all the discrepant results produced by assessments of youth behavior. Yet, these rater bias models inform the *usage assumptions* of the most widely implemented strategies for integrating multi-informant data. The term "usage assumptions" connotes any feature of an analytic procedure that a researcher accepts as a "true" or accurate fit to the data conditions within which the researcher implements the procedure (De Los Reyes et al., 2023a). In the case of implementing an integrative strategy, a user must accept as true the kinds of variance that the strategy models or treats as sources of valid data (De Los Reyes, 2024).

Rater bias models inform strategies that treat *common variance* as the key source of valid data—the variance shared among informants' reports (for a review, see Eid et al., 2008). Stated another way, the usage assumptions of strategies informed by rater bias models are as follows: Treat common variance as the only source of domain-relevant data about youth behavior and treat the informant-specific variance contained in discrepant results (i.e., *unique variance*) as *measurement confounds* such as random error and rater biases. Logically, if discrepant results are measurement confounds, then they reflect variance that is irrelevant to understanding behavioral domains (see also Millsap, 2011). Empirically, this means that measurement confounds cannot demonstrate valid relations to indices of behavioral domains (De Los Reyes, 2024).

As mentioned previously, rater bias models such as the depression→distortion hypothesis have played an influential role in how researchers have approached integrating data from multiple informants (for a review, see De Los Reyes & Epkins, 2023). For example, researchers often address discrepant results by taking an average or *composite score* among reports—a procedure that assumes the common variance is the only source of valid data among reports (e.g., Makol et al., 2020). More sophisticated approaches make similar assumptions regarding the relative value of common versus unique variance, such as constructing structural models focused on estimating common variance among reports (see Eid et al., 2008; Watts et al., 2022). Decision-making strategies for integrating data are not unique to working with large samples of multi-informant data. In fact, researchers routinely turn to using algorithms for integrating case-level multi-informant data to, for instance, determine the presence or absence of a level or set of behaviors (i.e., *AND/OR rules* in the case of diagnostic evaluations; see Baumgartner et al., 2021; Youngstrom et al., 2003). Some strategies eschew working with discrepant data altogether. For instance, the *primary outcome measure* procedure guides users to select one report a priori or in advance of conducting the assessment (see De Los Reyes et al., 2011). As another example, consider tests of measurement invariance, which are designed to remove item content that systematically differentiates informants' reports from each other (for a review, see De Los Reyes & Epkins, 2023). Taken together, despite the lack of compelling evidentiary support for rater bias models such as the depression→distortion hypothesis, they have nonetheless played a key role in guiding how scholars have integrated data from multiple informants.

1.3 Social Context Models and Falsifiability

In contrast to rater bias models, *social context models* hold that, under certain data conditions, discrepant results might contain domain-relevant information. The most frequently cited social context model is known as *situational specificity* (Achenbach et al., 1987). The notion of situational specificity holds that discrepant results are likely to occur when data conditions are characterized by two factors present in the assessment. First, the youth undergoing evaluation varies in how they behave within and across the social contexts in which they live day-to-day (e.g., home, school, community). Second, the assessment conducted to evaluate the youth's behavior involves collecting reports from structurally different informants. As with work informed by the depression→distortion hypothesis, decades of work on discrepant results have been informed by situational specificity and to interpret discrepancies in assessments of youth across periods of development (e.g., Bergold et al., 2019; Charamut et al., 2022; De Los Reyes et al., 2009, 2023a; Follet et al., 2023; Gresham et al., 1988, 2010; Kraemer et al., 2003; Larsson et al., 2000; McDermott et al., 2005; Ruffalo & Elliott, 1997; Szatmari et al., 1990). In this work, situational specificity has influenced the ways in which scholars have approached integrating data. Approaches informed by situational specificity extract valid data not only from what informants' reports share in common, but also what makes each of their reports unique (see De Los Reyes, 2024).

Three features of social context models distinguish them from rater bias models. First, social context models are informed by known data conditions. That is, they do not claim that all discrepant results are domain-relevant—just those that exist within a specific set of data conditions. In fact, this chapter describes a set of theoretical and methodological paradigms guided by social context models that are designed to distinguish domain-relevant discrepant results from those discrepancies that reflect measurement confounds. In this sense, social context models are *falsifiable* models—if they fail to explain or characterize the data conditions to which a user applies them, then the data will say so (see also Talbott et al., 2023).

Second, relative to rater bias models, far greater evidence supports social context models and their fit to the data conditions that typify assessments of youth behavior (for a review, see De Los Reyes et al., 2022b). We previously mentioned difficulties with falsifying or empirically probing interpretations of findings that researchers claim reflect support for the depression→distortion hypothesis. In contrast, a key element of research guided by social context models involves examining patterns of discrepant results among informants' reports produced within rigorously conducted validation studies. In the first of such studies, researchers characterized patterns of reports produced by parents and teachers in evaluations of disruptive behavior, including parent-teacher dyads who agreed in their reports of the child's behavior and dyads who disagreed in their reports (De Los Reyes et al., 2009). In this study, researchers also characterized children's behavior on a laboratory-controlled task of adult-child interactions and identified children who behaved disruptively across interactions with their parent and a non-parental adult, as well as children who behaved disruptively only with the parental adult and not the non-parental adult, and vice versa (Fig. 1.1). Patterns of parent-teacher reports predicted observed behavior, such that parents and teachers agreed in their reports when the child behaved disruptively across contexts and disagreed when children behaved disruptively within specific contexts. Domain-relevant patterns of parent-teacher reports have also been observed in assessments of youth autism, such that parent-teacher dyads show discernable patterns of agreement and disagreement (Fig. 1.2), and these patterns predict levels of severity of the youth's clinical presentation (Lerner et al., 2017). These findings are also not exclusive to characterizing patterns of reports among parents and teachers. For instance, in a large sample of adolescents receiving an evaluation at intake admission into an acute care facility, patterns of reports among parent-adolescent dyads exhibited a structure similar to the observed behavior depicted in Fig. 1.1 (see Fig. 1.3), and these patterns predicted characteristics of adolescents' acute care services (e.g., administration of standing antipsychotic medication and locked door seclusion; length of stay; Makol et al., 2019). Beyond these three studies, patterns of reports from structurally different informants have predicted a host of independent assessments of domains relevant to youth development (for a review, see De Los Reyes & Epkins, 2023), including (a) laboratory tests of pulmonary

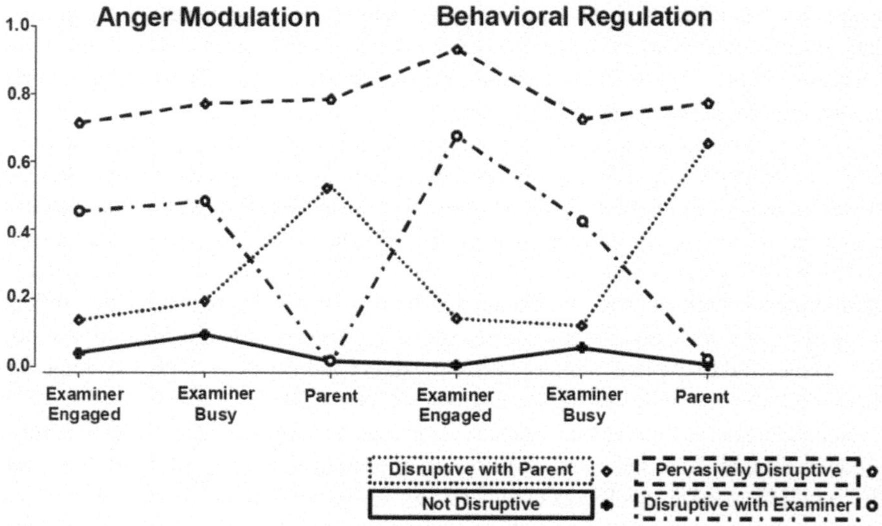

Fig. 1.1 Latent class solution of observed behavior on the Disruptive Behavior Diagnostic Observation Schedule. *Note*: The *x*-axis denotes the three measures of observed Anger Modulation and three measures of observed Behavioral Regulation across examiner-child interactions (when the examiner is either engaged or disengaged with the child) and parent-child interactions, respectively. The *y*-axis denotes the probability of observing high versus low levels of observed Anger Modulation and/or Behavioral Regulation. Latent classes are denoted via plotlines along the following classes of disruptive behavior: low disruptive behavior across interactions (Not Disruptive, $n = 153$), high disruptive behavior with parent only and not the clinical examiner (Disruptive with Parent, $n = 96$), high disruptive behavior with the clinical examiner only and not the parent (Disruptive with Examiner, $n = 49$), and high disruptive behavior with parent and clinical examiner (Pervasively Disruptive, $n = 29$). Reproduced from the figure used in the accepted manuscript version of De Los Reyes et al. (2009)

functioning (Al Ghriwati et al., 2018), (b) observed behavior during family interactions (De Los Reyes et al., 2016a), (c) observed behavior during classroom observations (De Los Reyes et al., 2022c), (d) clinical diagnoses (Becker-Haimes et al., 2018; Nichols & Tanner-Smith, 2022), (e) observed behavior during peer interactions (Charamut et al., 2022; Keeley et al., 2024), and (f) performance-based tasks of emotion recognition (e.g., De Los Reyes et al., 2013b).

Third, rater bias models and social context models each make distinct claims as to what discrepant results reflect. Consequently, these models guide users toward implementing different integrative strategies. Whereas the usage assumptions of strategies informed by rater bias models call for emphasizing common variance, social context models call for the use of integrative strategies that treat both common variance and unique variance as potential sources of valid or domain-relevant data. These models include (a) regression-based techniques that model discrepant results using statistical interactions (e.g., polynomial regression; Keeley et al., 2024), (b) person-centered techniques that capture qualitative differences in patterns of informants' reports (e.g., latent class analysis; Kang et al., 2023), and (c)

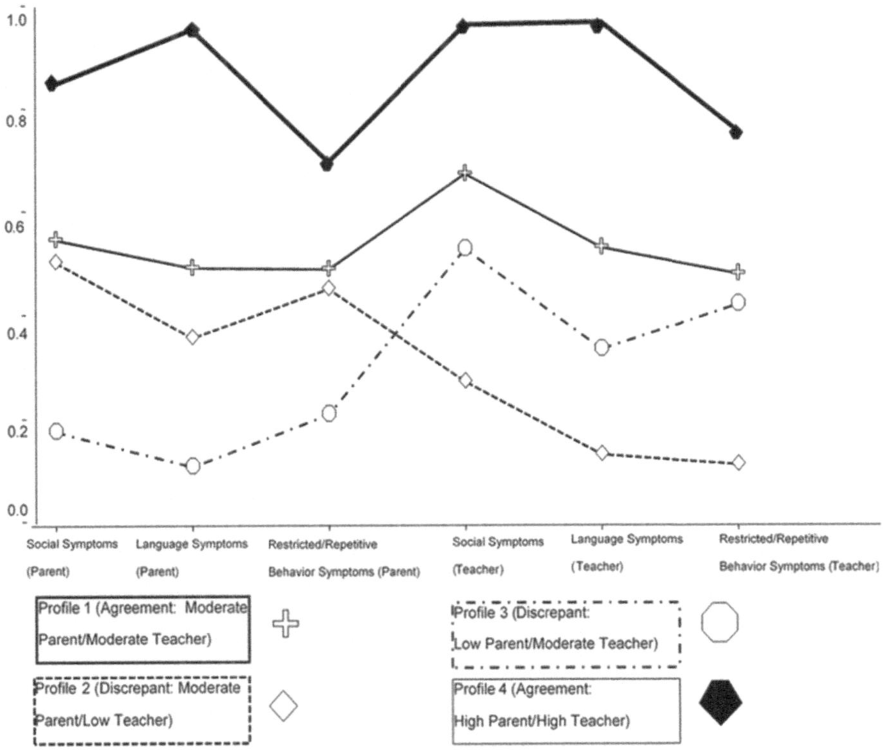

Fig. 1.2 Autism spectrum disorder (ASD) symptom severity informant agreement and discrepancy latent profiles. *Note*: Latent profiles of parent and teacher reports of ASD symptoms. Symptom ratings on the *x*-axis according to Child and Adolescent Symptom Inventory-4R. Standardized severity scores across these rating scales are on the *y*-axis. Profiles 1 and 4 represent cross-informant agreement (moderate and high severity ratings, respectively), whereas Profiles 2 and 3 represent cross-informant discrepancy (moderate parent/low teacher and moderate teacher/low parent severity ratings, respectively). Reproduced from the figure used in the accepted manuscript version of Lerner et al. (2017)

variable-centered techniques that decompose similarities and differences among reports into measured factor scores (e.g., principal components analysis; Charamut et al., 2022).

1.4 The Operations Triad Model and Conceptualizing Discrepant Results

Thus far, we have described tensions among three factors in scholarship in youth development: (a) available theories about discrepant results, (b) the evidence supporting these theories, and (c) the available strategies for integrating

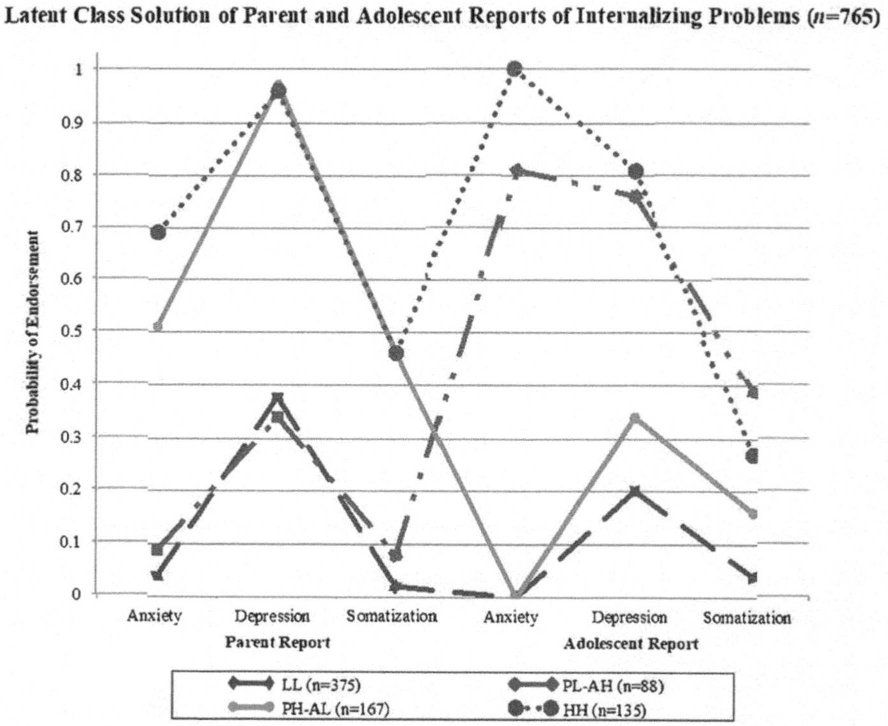

Fig. 1.3 Latent class solution of parent and adolescent reports of adolescent internalizing problems. *Note:* The *x*-axis denotes parent and adolescent internalizing problem reports, and the *y*-axis denotes the probability that informants reported clinically significant levels of internalizing problems. LL, parent-adolescent low; PL-AH, parent low-adolescent high; PHAL, parent high-adolescent low; HH, parent-adolescent high. Reproduced from the figure used in the accepted manuscript version of Makol et al. (2019)

multi-informant data. The persistence of these tensions creates barriers to developing guidelines for accurately interpreting discrepant results and integrating multi-informant data. The "origin story" for developing these guidelines lies with theory. Along these lines, in 2013, a theoretical framework emerged to facilitate conceptualizing discrepant results. A decade later, a validation paradigm emerged to guide empirical tests of these conceptualizations. This framework and the validation paradigm it inspired represent the conceptual and methodological foundations of this book. They also are the means through which this book resolves tensions in the literature surrounding integrating data from multiple informants and accurately assessing behavior in youth development.

The framework—*Operations Triad Model* (De Los Reyes, Thomas, et al., 2013a)—contains concepts to guide theorizing about the data conditions reflected by patterns of data produced by multi-informant reports of behavior (Fig. 1.4, Panels A–C). Importantly, the Operations Triad Model has been applied and/or adapted to a host of areas relevant to development across the lifespan, including (a)

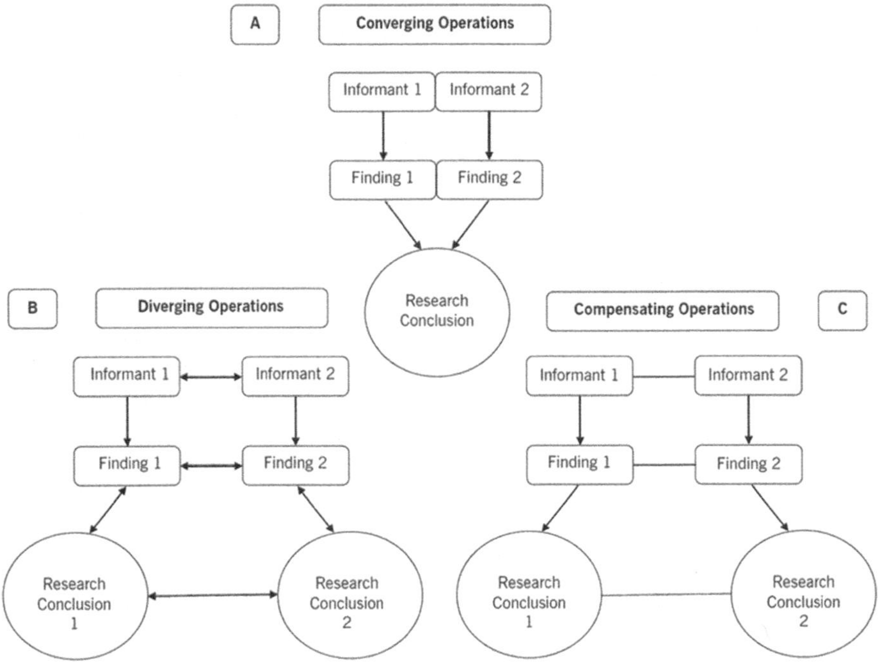

Fig. 1.4 Graphical representation of the research concepts that comprise the Operations Triad Model. The top half (**a**) represents Converging Operations: a set of measurement conditions for interpreting patterns of findings based on the consistency within which findings yield similar conclusions. The bottom half denotes two circumstances within which researchers identify discrepancies across empirical findings derived from multiple informants' reports and thus discrepancies in the research conclusions drawn from these reports. On the left (**b**) is a graphical representation of Diverging Operations: a set of measurement conditions for interpreting patterns of inconsistent findings based on hypotheses about variations in the behavior(s) assessed. The solid lines linking informants' reports, empirical findings derived from these reports, and conclusions based on empirical findings denote the systematic relations among these three study components. Further, the presence of dual arrowheads in the figure representing Diverging Operations conveys the idea that one ties meaning to the discrepancies among empirical findings and research conclusions and thus how one interprets informants' reports to vary as a function of variation in the behaviors being assessed. Lastly, on the right (**c**) is a graphical representation of Compensating Operations: a set of measurement conditions for interpreting patterns of inconsistent findings based on methodological features of the study's measures or informants. The dashed lines denote the lack of systematic relations among informants' reports, empirical findings, and research conclusions. Originally published in De Los Reyes et al. (2013a). © Annual Review of Clinical Psychology. Copyright 2012 Annual Reviews. All rights reserved. The Annual Reviews logo and other Annual Reviews products referenced herein are either registered trademarks or trademarks of Annual Reviews. All other marks are the property of their respective owner and/or licensor

education (Talbott et al., 2023), (b) special education (Casale & De Los Reyes, 2023; De Los Reyes et al., 2019c, 2022c; Genachowski et al., 2023; Talbott & De Los Reyes, 2022; von der Embse & De Los Reyes, 2024), (c) basic affective science (Kiel & Hummel, 2017), (d) psychophysiology (De Los Reyes & Aldao, 2015; De

Los Reyes et al., 2020), (e) family science (De Los Reyes & Ohannessian, 2016; De Los Reyes et al., 2013c, 2016b, 2019d; Hou et al., 2020; Kliewer et al., 2018; Korelitz & Garber, 2016; Nelemans et al., 2023; Ohannessian et al., 2016; Trang & Yates, 2020; Zhou et al., 2023), (f) adult mental health (De Los Reyes & Makol, 2021), (g) child welfare and maltreatment services (Makol et al., 2021; Romano et al., 2018), (h) suicide risk (Spears et al., 2023), and (i) the study of therapeutic processes (e.g., treatment fidelity and engagement; Lakind et al., 2022; McLeod et al., 2023). As such, the Operations Triad Model has wide applicability to behavioral assessments conducted by scholars in youth development.

Within the Operations Triad Model, *Compensating Operations* reflect data conditions in which discrepant results are best explained by measurement confounds (see Fig. 1.4, Panel C). Discrepant results that are explained by depression→distortion effects comprise one example of these confounds. Within these data conditions, optimizing measurement validity involves the use of integrative strategies that emphasize common variance (e.g., composite scoring, AND/OR rules).

The other two data conditions conceptualized within the Operations Triad Model reflect instances in which patterns of reports contain domain-relevant information. *Converging Operations* reflect data conditions in which each report yields the same conclusion as the other reports (see Fig. 1.4, Panel A). For example, informants' reports may converge if the informants observe youth behavior in the same context (e.g., two teachers rating the same youth) or observe youth in different contexts (e.g., parent vs. teacher) but rate a behavior that manifests persistently or severely across contexts (e.g., high levels of impairing hyperactivity at home and at school). In contrast, *Diverging Operations* reflects data conditions in which discrepant reports reflect valid variations in the behavior being assessed (see Fig. 1.4, Panel B). For instance, two informants' reports may diverge if the informants observe youth behavior in unique contexts (e.g., parent vs. teacher) and the youth behaves differently across contexts (e.g., hyperactivity at school but not home). Diverging Operations may also characterize youth who engage in a behavior that manifests covertly (e.g., symptoms of depression) in one context (e.g., with peers outside of the home) but not in another context (e.g., with parent at home). Here, Converging and Diverging Operations reflect data conditions that align with situational specificity.

1.5 Extending the Operations Triad Model to Inform Use of Integrative Strategies

A key implication of Converging and Diverging Operations is that if data conditions fit these concepts, then they inform the use of integrative strategies that preserve domain-relevant forms of both common and unique variance. Yet, in the years following the advent of the Operations Triad Model, researchers have repeatedly turned to addressing discrepant results using strategies that align with Compensating Operations (De Los Reyes & Epkins, 2023) and even when the discrepancies that researchers encounter may contain domain-relevant data (for a review, see De Los Reyes et al., 2022b). What this means is that merely conceptualizing discrepant results is insufficient. What we also require is a paradigm for directly testing the fit of integrative strategies to the data conditions in which researchers plan to implement them. The developers of the Operations Triad Model devised just such a paradigm, one that instantiates the framework's concepts in measurement—*Classifying Observations Necessitates Theory, Epistemology, and Testing* (*CONTEXT*; De Los Reyes et al., 2023a).

Using an innovative modification of traditional approaches to validation testing, users of CONTEXT take a hypothesis-driven approach to empirically testing patterns of multi-informant data and linking the findings of these tests to the concepts that underlie the Operations Triad Model. With CONTEXT, users go beyond conceptualizing that both Converging Operations and Diverging Operations scenarios might contain domain-relevant data. Users construct falsifiable tests of whether patterns of multi-informant reports contain domain-relevant data; these tests are guided by conceptually grounded hypotheses linked to Converging and Diverging Operations, such as situational specificity. Users of CONTEXT design measurement validation studies that leverage domain-relevant data from not only the instruments used in their studies, but also the structural differences among the informants completing the instruments. As such, users conduct falsifiable tests of a notion—that the structural differences among informants contain sources of valid data that, in combination with psychometrically sound responses to instrumentation, optimize measurement validity. Testing this notion involves characterizing patterns of the converging and/or discrepant results observed within multi-informant data and examining links between these patterns and validity criteria. Users of CONTEXT select validity criteria that are independent in modality from those used to collect informants' reports—behavioral observations, physiological readings, and performance on laboratory tasks, to name a few examples—but aligned with informants' reports in that the criteria reflect phenomena that are domain-relevant or pertinent to the content of reports provided by informants.

1.6 Concluding Comments

The Operations Triad Model and CONTEXT allow users to conduct fair, objective, and direct comparisons between competing strategies for integrating multi-informant data. As such, our larger goal involves comparing strategies informed by rater bias models on the one hand and social context models on the other. This larger goal informs a series of objectives. First, we provide an overview of two widely used integrative strategies—one informed by rater bias models (Chap. 2) and another informed by social context models (Chap. 3). Second, we describe research and theory on how the use of these two integrative strategies relates to the decisions researchers make when implementing them, namely, which data they input into their analytic models (i.e., number and kinds of informants; Chap. 4).

Third, this chapter cites work demonstrating that discrepant results generally appear when assessing domains of youth behavior. Yet, the strongest evidence for the validity of scores reflecting discrepant results comes from work about youth mental health domains (see De Los Reyes, 2024; De Los Reyes et al., 2023b). Thus, our two studies probe the validity performance of strategies for integrating multi-informant data about youth mental health. In Study 1 (Chap. 5), we construct Monte Carlo simulations of validity performance. We based these simulations on meta-analyses of discrepant results in youth mental health (i.e., Achenbach et al., 1987; De Los Reyes et al., 2015) and the latest work on the domain-relevant data that these discrepancies often contain (De Los Reyes & Epkins, 2023). Chapter 6 builds the rationale for subjecting integrative strategies to well-constructed tests of measurement validation, by describing key features of validity criteria in scholarship on youth development. Study 2 (Chap. 7) compares the criterion-related validity of these integrative strategies using a well-characterized study of adolescent mental health assessment. Fourth, we interpret our findings through the lenses of both rater bias and social context models; discuss their implications for theory, research, measurement, and applied work; and highlight key directions for future research (Chap. 8).

References

Achenbach, T. M. (2020). Bottom-up and top-down paradigms for psychopathology: A half century odyssey. *Annual Review of Clinical Psychology, 16*, 1–24. https://doi.org/10.1146/annurev-clinpsy-071119-115831

Achenbach, T. M., McConaughy, S. H., & Howell, C. T. (1987). Child/adolescent behavioral and emotional problems: Implications of cross-informant correlations for situational specificity. *Psychological Bulletin, 101*(2), 213–232. https://psycnet.apa.org/doi/10.1037/0033-2909.101.2.213

Achenbach, T. M., Krukowski, R. A., Dumenci, L., & Ivanova, M. Y. (2005). Assessment of adult psychopathology: Meta-analyses and implications of cross-informant correlations. *Psychological Bulletin, 131*(3), 361–382. https://psycnet.apa.org/doi/10.1037/0033-2909.131.3.361

Al Ghriwati, N., Winter, M. A., Greenlee, J. L., & Thompson, E. L. (2018). Discrepancies between parent and self-reports of adolescent psychosocial symptoms: Associations with family conflict and asthma outcomes. *Journal of Family Psychology, 32*(7), 992–997. https://doi.org/10.1037/fam0000459

Atkins, M. S., Cappella, E., Shernoff, E. S., Mehta, T. G., & Gustafson, E. L. (2017). Schooling and children's mental health: realigning resources to reduce disparities and advance public health. *Annual Review of Clinical Psychology, 13*, 123–147. https://doi.org/10.1146/annurev-clinpsy-032816-045234

Baumgartner, N., Foster, S., Emery, S., Berger, G., Walitza, S., & Häberling, I. (2021). How are discrepant parent–child reports integrated? A case of depressed adolescents. *Journal of Child and Adolescent Psychopharmacology, 31*(4), 279–287. https://doi.org/10.1089/cap.2020.0116

Becker-Haimes, E. M., Jensen-Doss, A., Birmaher, B., Kendall, P. C., & Ginsburg, G. S. (2018). Parent–youth informant disagreement: Implications for youth anxiety treatment. *Clinical Child Psychology and Psychiatry, 23*(1), 42–56. https://doi.org/10.1177/1359104516689586

Berg-Nielsen, T. S., Vika, A., & Dahl, A. A. (2003). When adolescents disagree with their mothers: CBCL-YSR discrepancies related to maternal depression and adolescent self-esteem. *Child: Care, Health and Development, 29*(3), 207–213. https://doi.org/10.1046/j.1365-2214.2003.00332.x

Berg-Nielsen, T. S., Solheim, E., Belsky, J., & Wichstrom, L. (2012). Preschoolers' psychosocial problems: In the eyes of the beholder? Adding teacher characteristics as determinants of discrepant parent–teacher reports. *Child Psychiatry and Human Development, 43*(3), 393–413. https://doi.org/10.1007/s10578-011-0271-0

Bergold, S., Christiansen, H., & Steinmayr, R. (2019). Interrater agreement and discrepancy when assessing problem behaviors, social-emotional skills, and developmental status of kindergarten children. *Journal of Clinical Psychology, 75*(12), 2210–2232. https://doi.org/10.1002/jclp.22840

Booth, C., Moreno-Agostino, D., & Fitzsimons, E. (2023). Parent-adolescent informant discrepancy on the Strengths and Difficulties Questionnaire in the UK Millennium Cohort Study. *Child and Adolescent Psychiatry and Mental Health, 17*(1), 57. https://doi.org/10.1186/s13034-023-00605-y

Boyle, M. H., & Pickles, A. R. (1997). Influence of maternal depressive symptoms on ratings of childhood behavior. *Journal of Abnormal Child Psychology, 25*(5), 399–412. https://doi.org/10.1023/A:1025737124888

Briggs-Gowan, M. J., Carter, A. S., & Schwab-Stone, M. (1996). Discrepancies among mother, child, and teacher reports: Examining the contributions of maternal depression and anxiety. *Journal of Abnormal Child Psychology, 24*(6), 749–765. https://doi.org/10.1007/BF01664738

Carlone, C., & Milan, S. (2021). Maternal depression and child externalizing behaviors: The role of attachment across development in low-income families. *Research on Child and Adolescent Psychopathology, 49*(5), 603–614. https://doi.org/10.1007/s10802-020-00747-z

Casale, G., & De Los Reyes, A. (2023). An integrated model for school-based mental health assessment in inclusive classrooms. *Empirische Sonderpädagogik [Empirical Special Education]., 15*(3), 214–233. https://doi.org/10.2440/003-0008. https://psycnet.apa.org/doi/10.1037/0012-1649.40.2.149

Castagna, P. J., Lilly, M. E., & Davis, T. E. I. I. I. (2020). Maternal reporting of child psychopathology: The effect of defensive responding. *Current Psychology: A Journal for Diverse Perspectives on Diverse Psychological Issues, 39*(1), 315–324. https://doi.org/10.1007/s12144-017-9765-7

Charamut, N. R., Racz, S. J., Wang, M., & De Los Reyes, A. (2022). Integrating multi-informant reports of youth mental health: A construct validation test of Kraemer and Colleagues' (2003) Satellite Model. *Frontiers in Psychology, 13*, 911629. https://doi.org/10.3389/fpsyg.2022.911629

Chi, T. C., & Hinshaw, S. P. (2002). Mother-child relationships of children with ADHD: The role of maternal depressive symptoms and depression-related distortions. *Journal of Abnormal Child Psychology, 30*(4), 387–400. https://doi.org/10.1023/A:1015770025043

Chilcoat, H. D., & Breslau, N. (1997). Does psychiatric history bias mothers' reports? An application of a new analytic approach. *Journal of the American Academy of Child and Adolescent Psychiatry, 36*(7), 971–979. https://doi.org/10.1097/00004583-199707000-00020

Cicchetti, D. (1984). The emergence of developmental psychopathology. *Child Development, 55*(1), 1–7. https://doi.org/10.2307/1129830

Clarkson, T., Kang, E., Capriola-Hall, N., Lerner, M. D., Jarcho, J., & Prinstein, M. J. (2020). Meta-analysis of the RDoC social processing domain across units of analysis in children and adolescents. *Journal of Clinical Child and Adolescent Psychology, 49*(3), 297–321. https://doi.org/10.1080/15374416.2019.1678167

De Los Reyes, A. (2011). More than measurement error: Discovering meaning behind informant discrepancies in clinical assessments of children and adolescents. *Journal of Clinical Child and Adolescent Psychology, 40*(1), 1–9. https://doi.org/10.1080/15374416.2011.533405
De Los Reyes, A. (2024). *Discrepant results in mental health research: What they mean, why they matter, and how they inform scientific practices.* Oxford University Press.
De Los Reyes, A., & Aldao, A. (2015). Introduction to the special issue. Toward implementing physiological measures in clinical child and adolescent assessments. *Journal of Clinical Child and Adolescent Psychology, 44*(2), 221–237. https://doi.org/10.1080/15374416.2014.891227
De Los Reyes, A., & Epkins, C. C. (2023). Introduction to the special issue. A dozen years of demonstrating that informant discrepancies are more than measurement error: Toward guidelines for integrating data from multi-informant assessments of youth mental health. *Journal of Clinical Child and Adolescent Psychology, 52*(1), 1–18. https://doi.org/10.1080/15374416.2022.2158843
De Los Reyes, A., & Kazdin, A. E. (2005). Informant discrepancies in the assessment of childhood psychopathology: A critical review, theoretical framework, and recommendations for further study. *Psychological Bulletin, 131*(4), 483–509. https://doi.org/10.1037/0033-2909.131.4.483
De Los Reyes, A., & Kazdin, A. E. (2006). Conceptualizing changes in behavior in intervention research: The range of possible changes model. *Psychological Review, 113*(3), 554–583. https://doi.org/10.1037/0033-295X.113.3.554
De Los Reyes, A., & Kazdin, A. E. (2008). When the evidence says, "Yes, no, and maybe so": Attending to and interpreting inconsistent findings among evidence-based interventions. *Current Directions in Psychological Science, 17*(1), 47–51. https://doi.org/10.1111/j.1467-8721.2008.00546.x
De Los Reyes, A., & Makol, B. A. (2021). Interpreting convergences and divergences in multi-informant, multi-method assessment. In J. Mihura (Ed.), *The Oxford handbook of personality and psychopathology assessment* (2nd ed.). Oxford. Advance online publication. https://doi.org/10.1093/oxfordhb/9780190092689.013.33
De Los Reyes, A., & Makol, B. A. (2022). Informant reports in clinical assessment. In G. Asmundson (Ed.), *Comprehensive clinical psychology* (Vol. 4, 2nd ed., pp. 105–122). Elsevier. https://doi.org/10.1016/B978-0-12-818697-8.00113-8
De Los Reyes, A., & Ohannessian, C. M. (2016). Introduction to the special issue. Discrepancies in adolescent-parent perceptions of the family and adolescent adjustment. *Journal of Youth and Adolescence, 45*(10), 1957–1972. https://doi.org/10.1007/s10964-016-0533-z
De Los Reyes, A., & Prinstein, M. J. (2004). Applying depression-distortion hypotheses to the assessment of peer victimization in adolescents. *Journal of Clinical Child and Adolescent Psychology, 33*(2), 325–335. https://doi.org/10.1207/s15374424jccp3302_14
De Los Reyes, A., Goodman, K. L., Kliewer, W., & Reid-Quiñones, K. (2008). Whose depression relates to discrepancies? Testing relations between informant characteristics and informant discrepancies from both informants' perspectives. *Psychological Assessment, 20*(2), 139–149. https://doi.org/10.1037/1040-3590.20.2.139
De Los Reyes, A., Henry, D. B., Tolan, P. H., & Wakschlag, L. S. (2009). Linking informant discrepancies to observed variations in young children's disruptive behavior. *Journal of Abnormal Child Psychology, 37*(5), 637–652. https://doi.org/10.1007/s10802-009-9307-3
De Los Reyes, A., Kundey, S. M. A., & Wang, M. (2011). The end of the primary outcome measure: A research agenda for constructing its replacement. *Clinical Psychology Review, 31*(5), 829–838. https://doi.org/10.1016/j.cpr.2011.03.011
De Los Reyes, A., Thomas, S. A., Goodman, K. L., & Kundey, S. M. A. (2013a). Principles underlying the use of multiple informants' reports. *Annual Review of Clinical Psychology, 9*, 123–149. https://doi.org/10.1146/annurev-clinpsy-050212-185617
De Los Reyes, A., Lerner, M. D., Thomas, S. A., Daruwala, S. E., & Goepel, K. A. (2013b). Discrepancies between parent and adolescent beliefs about daily life topics and performance on an emotion recognition task. *Journal of Abnormal Child Psychology, 41*(6), 971–982. https://doi.org/10.1007/s10802-013-9733-0

De Los Reyes, A., Salas, S., Menzer, M. M., & Daruwala, S. E. (2013c). Criterion validity of interpreting scores from multi-informant statistical interactions as measures of informant discrepancies in psychological assessments of children and adolescents. *Psychological Assessment, 25*(2), 509–519. https://doi.org/10.1037/a0032081

De Los Reyes, A., Augenstein, T. M., Wang, M., Thomas, S. A., Drabick, D. A. G., Burgers, D., & Rabinowitz, J. (2015). The validity of the multi-informant approach to assessing child and adolescent mental health. *Psychological Bulletin, 141*(4), 858–900. https://doi.org/10.1037/a0038498

De Los Reyes, A., Alfano, C. A., Lau, S., Augenstein, T. M., & Borelli, J. L. (2016a). Can we use convergence between caregiver reports of adolescent mental health to index severity of adolescent mental health concerns? *Journal of Child and Family Studies, 25*(1), 109–123. https://doi.org/10.1007/s10826-015-0216-5

De Los Reyes, A., Ohannessian, C. M., & Laird, R. D. (2016b). Developmental changes in discrepancies between adolescents' and their mothers' views of family communication. *Journal of Child and Family Studies, 25*(3), 790–797. https://doi.org/10.1007/s10826-015-0275-7

De Los Reyes, A., Augenstein, T. M., & Aldao, A. (2017). Assessment issues in child and adolescent psychotherapy. In J. R. Weisz & A. E. Kazdin (Eds.), *Evidence-based psychotherapies for children and adolescents* (3rd ed., pp. 537–554). Guilford.

De Los Reyes, A., Ohannessian, C. M., & Racz, S. J. (2019a). Discrepancies between adolescent and parent reports about family relationships. *Child Development Perspectives, 13*(1), 53–58. https://doi.org/10.1111/cdep.12306

De Los Reyes, A., Lerner, M. D., Keeley, L. M., Weber, R. J., Drabick, D. A., Rabinowitz, J., & Goodman, K. L. (2019b). Improving interpretability of subjective assessments about psychological phenomena: a review and cross-cultural meta-analysis. *Review of General Psychology, 23*(3), 293–319. https://doi.org/10.1177/1089268019837645

De Los Reyes, A., Cook, C. R., Gresham, F. M., Makol, B. A., & Wang, M. (2019c). Informant discrepancies in assessments of psychosocial functioning in school-based services and research: Review and directions for future research. *Journal of School Psychology, 74*, 74–89. https://doi.org/10.1016/j.jsp.2019.05.005

De Los Reyes, A., Makol, B. A., Racz, S. J., Youngstrom, E. A., Lerner, M. D., & Keeley, L. M. (2019d). The Work and Social Adjustment Scale for Youth: A measure for assessing youth psychosocial impairment regardless of mental health status. *Journal of Child and Family Studies, 28*(1), 1–16. https://doi.org/10.1007/s10826-018-1238-6

De Los Reyes, A., Drabick, D. A. G., Makol, B. A., & Jakubovic, R. (2020). Introduction to the special section: The Research Domain Criteria's units of analysis and cross-unit correspondence in youth mental health research. *Journal of Clinical Child and Adolescent Psychology, 49*(3), 279–296. https://doi.org/10.1080/15374416.2020.1738238

De Los Reyes, A., Talbott, E., Power, T., Michel, J., Cook, C. R., Racz, S. J., & Fitzpatrick, O. (2022a). The Needs-to-Goals Gap: How informant discrepancies in youth mental health assessments impact service delivery. *Clinical Psychology Review, 92*, Article 102114. https://doi.org/10.1016/j.cpr.2021.102114

De Los Reyes, A., Tyrell, F. A., Watts, A. L., & Asmundson, G. J. G. (2022b). Conceptual, methodological, and measurement factors that disqualify use of measurement invariance techniques to detect informant discrepancies in youth mental health assessments. *Frontiers in Psychology, 13*, Article 931296. https://doi.org/10.3389/fpsyg.2022.931296

De Los Reyes, A., Cook, C. R., Sullivan, M., Morrell, N., Hamlin, C., Wang, M., Gresham, F. M., Makol, B. A., Keeley, L. M., & Qasmieh, N. (2022c). The Work and Social Adjustment Scale for Youth: Psychometric properties of the teacher version and evidence of contextual variability in psychosocial impairments. *Psychological Assessment, 34*(8), 777–790. https://doi.org/10.1037/pas0001139

De Los Reyes, A., Wang, M., Lerner, M. D., Makol, B. A., Fitzpatrick, O., & Weisz, J. R. (2023a). The Operations Triad Model and youth mental health assessments: Catalyzing a paradigm shift in measurement validation. *Journal of Clinical Child and Adolescent Psychology, 52*(1), 19–54. https://doi.org/10.1080/15374416.2022.2111684

De Los Reyes, A., Epkins, C. C., Asmundson, G. J. G., Augenstein, T. M., Becker, K. D., Becker, S. P., Bonadio, F. T., Borelli, J. L., Boyd, R. C., Bradshaw, C. P., Burns, G. L., Casale, G., Causadias, J. M., Cha, C. B., Chorpita, B. F., Cohen, J. R., Comer, J. S., Crowell, S. E., Dirks, M. A., et al. (2023b). Editorial statement about *JCCAP*'s 2023 special issue on informant discrepancies in youth mental health assessments: Observations, guidelines, and future directions grounded in 60 years of research. *Journal of Clinical Child and Adolescent Psychology, 52*(1), 147–158. https://doi.org/10.1080/15374416.2022.2158842

Durbin, C. E., & Wilson, S. (2012). Convergent validity of and bias in maternal reports of child emotion. *Psychological Assessment, 24*(3), 647–660. https://doi.org/10.1037/a0026607

Eid, M., Nussbeck, F. W., Geiser, C., Cole, D. A., Gollwitzer, M., & Lischetzke, T. (2008). Structural equation modeling of multitrait-multimethod data: Different models for different types of methods. *Psychological Methods, 13*(3), 230–253. https://doi.org/10.1037/a0013219

Follet, L., Okuno, H., & De Los Reyes, A. (2023). Assessing peer-related impairments linked to adolescent social anxiety: Strategic selection of informants optimizes prediction of clinically relevant domains. *Behavior Therapy, 54*(1), 29–42. https://doi.org/10.1016/j.beth.2022.06.010

Gartstein, M. A., Bridgett, D. J., Dishion, T. J., & Kaufman, N. K. (2009). Depressed mood and maternal report of child behavior problems: Another look at the depression-distortion hypothesis. *Journal of Applied Developmental Psychology, 30*(2), 149–160. https://doi.org/10.1016/j.appdev.2008.12.001

Genachowski, K. J., Starin, N. S., Cummings, C. M., Alvord, M. K., & Rich, B. A. (2023). Interpretation of informant discrepancy in school-based psychological assessment of internalizing and externalizing symptoms. *Journal of Emotional and Behavioral Disorders, 31*(4), 248–259. https://doi.org/10.1177/10634266221119742

Goodman, S. H., Simon, H. F. M., Shamblaw, A. L., & Kim, C. Y. (2020). Parenting as a mediator of associations between depression in mothers and children's functioning: A systematic review and meta-analysis. *Clinical Child and Family Psychology Review, 23*(4), 427–460. https://doi.org/10.1007/s10567-020-00322-4

Gresham, F. M., Evans, S., & Elliott, S. N. (1988). Academic and social self-efficacy scale: development and initial validation. *Journal of Psychoeducational Assessment, 6*(2), 125–138. https://doi.org/10.1177/073428298800600204

Gresham, F. M., Elliott, S. N., Cook, C. R., Vance, M. J., & Kettler, R. (2010). Cross-informant agreement for ratings for social skill and problem behavior ratings: An investigation of the Social Skills Improvement System—Rating Scales. *Psychological Assessment, 22*(1), 157–166. https://doi.org/10.1037/a0018124

Haeffel, G. J., Jeronimus, B. F., Kaiser, B. N., Weaver, L. J., Soyster, P. D., Fisher, A. J., Vargas, I., Goodson, J. T., & Lu, W. (2022). Folk classification and factor rotations: Whales, Sharks, and the problems with the Hierarchical Taxonomy of Psychopathology (HiTOP). *Clinical Psychological Science, 10*(2), 259–278. https://doi.org/10.1177/21677026211002500

Hawker, D. S., & Boulton, M. J. (2000). Twenty years' research on peer victimization and psychosocial maladjustment: A meta-analytic review of cross-sectional studies. *The Journal of Child Psychology and Psychiatry and Allied Disciplines, 41*(4), 441–455. https://doi.org/10.1111/1469-7610.00629

Hendriks, A. M., Van der Giessen, D., Stams, G. J. J. M., & Overbeek, G. (2018). The association between parent-reported and observed parenting: A multi-level meta-analysis. *Psychological Assessment, 30*(5), 621–633. https://doi.org/10.1037/pas0000500

Hou, Y., Benner, A. D., Kim, S. Y., Chen, S., Spitz, S., Shi, Y., & Beretvas, T. (2020). Discordance in parents' and adolescents' reports of parenting: A meta-analysis and qualitative review. *American Psychologist, 75*(3), 329–348. https://doi.org/10.1037/amp0000463

Hunsley, J., & Mash, E. J. (2007). Evidence-based assessment. *Annual Review of Clinical Psychology, 3*, 29–51. https://doi.org/10.1146/annurev.clinpsy.3.022806.091419

Ivanova, M., Achenbach, T. M., & Turner, L. (2022). Associations of parental depression with children's internalizing and externalizing: Meta-analyses of cross-sectional and longitudinal effects. *Journal of Clinical Child and Adolescent Psychology, 51*(6), 827–849. https://doi.org/10.1080/15374416.2022.2127104

Kagan, J., Snidman, N., McManis, M., Woodward, S., & Hardway, C. (2002). One measure, one meaning: Multiple measures, clearer meaning. *Development and Psychopathology, 14*(3), 463–475. https://doi.org/10.1017/S0954579402003048

Kang, E., Lerner, M. D., & Gadow, K. D. (2023). The importance of parent-teacher informant discrepancy in characterizing autistic youth: A replication latent profile analysis. *Journal of Clinical Child and Adolescent Psychology, 52*(1), 108–118. https://doi.org/10.1080/15374416.2022.2154217

Kaurin, A., Sequeira, S. L., Ladouceur, C. D., McKone, K. M. P., Rosen, D., Jones, N., Wright, A. G. C., & Silk, J. S. (2022). Modeling sensitivity to social threat in adolescent girls: A psychoneurometric approach. *Journal of Psychopathology and Clinical Science, 131*(6), 641–652. https://doi.org/10.1037/abn0000532

Keeley, L. M., Laird, R. D., Qasmieh, N., Racz, S. J., Ohannessian, C. M., & De Los Reyes, A. (2024). When parents and adolescents make discrepant reports about parental monitoring: Links to adolescent anxiety when interacting with unfamiliar peers. *Journal of Psychopathology and Behavioral Assessment, 46*(2), 343–356. https://doi.org/10.1007/s10862-024-10132-5

Kiel, E. J., & Hummel, A. C. (2017). Contextual influences on concordance between maternal report and laboratory observation of toddler fear. *Emotion, 17*(2), 240–250. https://doi.org/10.1037/emo0000230

Kliewer, W., Sosnowski, D. W., Wilkins, S., Garr, K., Booth, C., McGuire, K., & Wright, A. W. (2018). Do parent-adolescent discrepancies predict deviant peer affiliation and subsequent substance use? *Journal of Youth and Adolescence, 47*(12), 2596–2607. https://doi.org/10.1007/s10964-018-0879-5

Korelitz, K. E., & Garber, J. (2016). Congruence of parents' and children's perceptions of parenting: A meta-analysis. *Journal of Youth and Adolescence, 45*(10), 1973–1995. https://doi.org/10.1007/s10964-016-0524-0

Kraemer, H. C., Measelle, J. R., Ablow, J. C., Essex, M. J., Boyce, W. T., & Kupfer, D. J. (2003). A new approach to integrating data from multiple informants in psychiatric assessment and research: Mixing and matching contexts and perspectives. *American Journal of Psychiatry, 160*(9), 1566–1577. https://doi.org/10.1176/appi.ajp.160.9.1566

Kroes, G., Veerman, J. W., & De Bruyn, E. E. J. (2003). Bias in parental reports? Maternal psychopathology and the reporting of problem behavior in clinic-referred children. *European Journal of Psychological Assessment, 19*(3), 195–203. https://doi.org/10.1027/1015-5759.19.3.195

Lakind, D., Bradley, W. J., Patel, A., Chorpita, B. F., & Becker, K. D. (2022). A multidimensional examination of the measurement of treatment engagement: Implications for children's mental health services and research. *Journal of Clinical Child and Adolescent Psychology, 51*(4), 453–468. https://doi.org/10.1080/15374416.2021.1941057

Larsson, B., Melin, L., & Morris, R. J. (2000). Anxiety in Swedish school children: Situational specificity, informant variability and coping strategies. *Scandinavian Journal of Behaviour Therapy, 29*(3–4), 127–139. https://doi.org/10.1080/028457100300049755

Lerner, M. D., De Los Reyes, A., Drabick, D. G., Gerber, A. H., & Gadow, K. D. (2017). Informant discrepancy defines discrete, clinically useful autism spectrum disorder subgroups. *Journal of Child Psychology and Psychiatry, 58*(7), 829–839. https://doi.org/10.1111/jcpp.12730

Luthar, S. S., Cicchetti, D., & Becker, B. (2000). The construct of resilience: A critical evaluation and guidelines for future work. *Child Development, 71*(3), 543–562. https://doi.org/10.1111/1467-8624.00164

Madsen, K. B., Rask, C. U., Olsen, J., Niclasen, J., & Obel, C. (2020). Depression-related distortions in maternal reports of child behaviour problems. *European Child and Adolescent Psychiatry, 29*(3), 275–285. https://doi.org/10.1007/s00787-019-01351-3

Makol, B. A., De Los Reyes, A., Ostrander, R., & Reynolds, E. K. (2019). Parent-youth divergence (and convergence) in reports of youth internalizing problems in psychiatric inpatient care. *Journal of Abnormal Child Psychology, 47*(10), 1677–1689. https://doi.org/10.1007/s10802-019-00540-7

Makol, B. A., Youngstrom, E. A., Racz, S. J., Qasmieh, N., Glenn, L. E., & De Los Reyes, A. (2020). Integrating multiple informants' reports: How conceptual and measurement models may address long-standing problems in clinical decision-making. *Clinical Psychological Science, 8*(6), 953–970. https://doi.org/10.1177/2167702620924439

Makol, B. A., De Los Reyes, A., Garrido, E., Harlaar, N., & Taussig, H. (2021). Assessing the mental health of maltreated youth with child welfare involvement using multi-informant reports. *Child Psychiatry and Human Development, 52*(1), 49–62. https://doi.org/10.1007/s10578-020-00985-8

McDermott, P. A., Steinberg, C. M., & Angelo, L. E. (2005). Situational specificity makes the difference in assessment of youth behavior disorders. *Psychology in the Schools, 42*(2), 121–136. https://doi.org/10.1002/pits.20050

McLeod, B. D., Porter, N., Hogue, A., Becker-Haimes, E., & Jensen-Doss, A. (2023). What is the status of multi-informant treatment fidelity research? *Journal of Clinical Child and Adolescent Psychology, 52*(1), 74–94. https://doi.org/10.1080/15374416.2022.2151713

Meyer, G. J., Finn, S. E., Eyde, L. D., Kay, G. G., Moreland, K. L., Dies, R. R., Eisman, E. J., Kubiszyn, T. W., & Reed, G. M. (2001). Psychological testing and psychological assessment: A review of evidence and issues. *American Psychologist, 56*(2), 128–165. https://doi.org/10.1037/0003-066X.56.2.128

Millsap, E. (2011). *Statistical methods for studying measurement invariance*. Taylor and Francis.

Müller, J. M., & Furniss, T. (2013). Correction of distortions in distressed mothers' ratings of their preschool children's psychopathology. *Psychiatry Research, 210*(1), 294–301. https://doi.org/10.1016/j.psychres.2013.03.025

Müller, J. M., Romer, G., & Achtergarde, S. (2014). Correction of distortion in distressed mothers' ratings of their preschool-aged children's Internalizing and Externalizing scale score. *Psychiatry Research, 215*(1), 170–175. https://doi.org/10.1016/j.psychres.2013.10.035

Najman, J. M., Williams, G. M., Nikles, J., Spence, S., Bor, W., O'Callaghan, M., Le Brocque, R., & Andersen, M. J. (2000). Mothers' mental illness and child behavior problems: Cause–effect association or observation bias? *Journal of the American Academy of Child and Adolescent Psychiatry, 39*(5), 592–602. https://doi.org/10.1097/00004583-200005000-00013

Nelemans, S. A., Mastrotheodoros, S., Çiftçi, L., Meeus, W., & Branje, S. (2023). Do you see what I see? Longitudinal associations between mothers' and adolescents' perceptions of their relationship and adolescent internalizing symptoms. *Research on Child and Adolescent Psychopathology, 51*(2), 177–192. https://doi.org/10.1007/s10802-022-00975-5

Nichols, L. M., & Tanner-Smith, E. E. (2022). Discrepant parent-adolescent reports of parenting practices: Associations with adolescent internalizing and externalizing symptoms. *Journal of Youth and Adolescence, 51*(6), 1153–1168. https://doi.org/10.1007/s10964-022-01601-9

Ohannessian, C. M., Laird, R. D., & De Los Reyes, A. (2016). Discrepancies in adolescents' and their mother's perceptions of the family and mothers' psychological symptomatology. *Journal of Youth and Adolescence, 45*(10), 2011–2021. https://doi.org/10.1007/s10964-016-0477-3

Olino, T. M., Guerra-Guzman, K., Hayden, E. P., & Klein, D. N. (2020). Evaluating maternal psychopathology biases in reports of child temperament: An investigation of measurement invariance. *Psychological Assessment, 32*(11), 1037–1046. https://doi.org/10.1037/pas0000945

Olino, T. M., Michelini, G., Mennies, R. J., Kotov, R., & Klein, D. N. (2021). Does maternal psychopathology bias reports of offspring symptoms? A study using moderated non-linear factor analysis. *Journal of Child Psychology and Psychiatry, 62*(10), 1195–1201. https://doi.org/10.1111/jcpp.13394

Phares, V., & Hankinson, J. (2020). Evidence-based assessment and measurement-based care. In *Handbook of evidence-based therapies for children and adolescents: Bridging science and practice* (pp. 25–38). Springer.

Renk, K., & Phares, V. (2004). Cross-informant ratings of social competence in children and adolescents. *Clinical Psychology Review, 24*, 239–254. https://doi.org/10.1016/j.cpr.2004.01.004

Rescorla, L. A., Ginzburg, S., Achenbach, T. M., Ivanova, M. Y., Almqvist, F., Begovac, I., et al. (2013). Cross-informant agreement between parent-reported and adolescent self-reported problems in 25 societies. *Journal of Clinical Child and Adolescent Psychology, 42*(2), 262–273. https://doi.org/10.1080/15374416.2012.717870

Rescorla, L. A., Ewing, G., Ivanova, M. Y., Aebi, M., Bilenberg, N., Dieleman, G. C., et al. (2017). Parent–adolescent cross-informant agreement in clinically referred samples: findings from seven societies. *Journal of Clinical Child and Adolescent Psychology, 46*(1), 74–87. https://doi.org/10.1080/15374416.2016.1266642

Richters, J. E. (1992). Depressed mothers as informants about their children: A critical review of the evidence for distortion. *Psychological Bulletin, 112*(3), 485–499. https://doi.org/10.1037/0033-2909.112.3.485

Romano, E., Weegar, K., Babchishin, L., & Saini, M. (2018). Cross-informant agreement on mental health outcomes in children with maltreatment histories: A systematic review. *Psychology of Violence, 8*(1), 19–30. https://doi.org/10.1037/vio0000086

Ruffalo, S. L., & Elliott, S. N. (1997). Teachers' and parents' ratings of children's social skills: A closer look at cross-informant agreements through an item analysis protocol. *School Psychology Review, 26*(3), 489–501. https://doi.org/10.1080/02796015.1997.12085882

Spears, A. P., Gratch, I., Nam, R. J., Goger, P., & Cha, C. B. (2023). Future directions in understanding and interpreting discrepant reports of suicidal thoughts and behaviors among youth. *Journal of Clinical Child & Adolescent Psychology, 52*(1), 134–146. https://doi.org/10.1080/15374416.2022.2145567

Stratis, E. A., & Lecavalier, L. (2015). Informant agreement for youth with autism spectrum disorder or intellectual disability: A meta-analysis. *Journal of Autism and Developmental Disorders, 45*(4), 1026–1041. https://doi.org/10.1007/s10803-014-2258-8

Sudkamp, A., Kaiser, J., & Moller, J. (2012). Accuracy of teachers' judgments of students' academic achievement: A meta-analysis. *Journal of Educational Psychology, 104*(3), 743–762. https://doi.org/10.1037/a0027627

Szatmari, P., Offord, D. R., Siegel, L. S., Finlayson, M. A., & Tuff, L. (1990). The clinical significance of neurocognitive impairments among children with psychiatric disorders: Diagnosis and situational specificity. *Child Psychology and Psychiatry and Allied Disciplines, 31*(2), 287–299. https://doi.org/10.1111/j.1469-7610.1990.tb01567.x

Talbott, E., & De Los Reyes, A. (2022). Making sense of multiple data sources: Using single case design research for behavioral decision making. In T. Farmer, E. Talbott, K. McMaster, D. Lee, & T. Aceves (Eds.), *Handbook of special education research: Theory, methods, and developmental processes* (pp. 231–244). Routledge.

Talbott, E., De Los Reyes, A., Kearns, D. M., Mancilla-Martinez, J., Cook, C. R., & Wang, M. (2023). Evidence-based assessment in special education research: Advancing the use of evidence in assessment tools and empirical processes. *Exceptional Children, 89*(4), 467–487. https://doi.org/10.1177/00144029231171092

Trang, D. T., & Yates, T. M. (2020). (In)congruent parent–child reports of parental behaviors and later child outcomes. *Journal of Child and Family Studies, 29*(7), 1845–1860. https://doi.org/10.1007/s10826-020-01733-1

Treutler, C. M., & Epkins, C. C. (2003). Are discrepancies among child, mother, and father reports on children's behavior related to parents' psychological symptoms and aspects of parent-child relationships? *Journal of Abnormal Child Psychology, 31*(1), 13–27. https://doi.org/10.1023/A:1021765114434

von der Embse, N., & De Los Reyes, A. (2024). Advancing equity in access to school mental health through multiple informant decision-making. *Journal of School Psychology, 104*, 101310. https://doi.org/10.1016/j.jsp.2024.101310

Watts, A. L., Makol, B. A., Palumbo, I. M., De Los Reyes, A., Olino, T. M., Latzman, R. D., DeYoung, C. G., Wood, P. K., & Sher, K. J. (2022). How robust is the p-factor? Using multitrait-multimethod modeling to inform the meaning of general factors of psychopathology in youth. *Clinical Psychological Science, 10*(4), 640–661. https://doi.org/10.1177/21677026211055170

Weisz, J. R., Doss, A. J., & Hawley, K. M. (2005). Youth psychotherapy outcome research: A review and critique of the evidence base. *Annual Review of Psychology, 56*, 337–363. https://doi.org/10.1146/annurev.psych.55.090902.141449

Wesselhoeft, R., Davidsen, K., Sibbersen, C., Kyhl, H., Talati, A., Andersen, M. S., & Bilenberg, N. (2021). Maternal prenatal stress and postnatal depressive symptoms: Discrepancy between mother and teacher reports of toddler psychological problems. *Social Psychiatry and Psychiatric Epidemiology, 56*(4), 559–570. https://doi.org/10.1007/s00127-020-01964-z

Wright, A. J., Pade, H., Gottfried, E. D., Arbisi, P. A., McCord, D. M., & Wygant, D. B. (2022). Evidence-based clinical psychological assessment (EBCPA): Review of current state of the literature and best practices. *Professional Psychology: Research and Practice, 53*(4), 372–386. https://doi.org/10.1037/pro0000447

Youngstrom, E. A., & Van Meter, A. (2016). Empirically supported assessment of children and adolescents. *Clinical Psychology: Science and Practice, 23*(4), 327–347. https://doi.org/10.1111/cpsp.1217

Youngstrom, E. A., Izard, C., & Ackerman, B. (1999). Dysphoria-related bias in maternal ratings of children. *Journal of Consulting and Clinical Psychology, 67*(6), 905–916. https://doi.org/10.1037/0022-006X.67.6.905

Youngstrom, E. A., Findling, R. L., & Calabrese, J. R. (2003). Who are the comorbid adolescents? Agreement between psychiatric diagnosis, youth, parent, and teacher report. *Journal of Abnormal Child Psychology, 31*(3), 231–245. https://doi.org/10.1023/A:1023244512119

Zhou, Y., Qu, D., Xu, C., Zhang, Q., & Yu, N. X. (2023). How does (in)congruence in perceived adolescent–parent closeness link to adolescent socioemotional well-being? The mediating role of resilience. *Journal of Happiness Studies, 24*(2), 839–856. https://doi.org/10.1007/s10902-023-00624-8

Chapter 2
Strategies for Integrating Behavioral Data: Rater Bias Models of Youth Development

Chapters 2 and 3 review how researchers have implemented strategies for integrating multi-informant data when assessing youth behavior. It is beyond the scope of this book to exhaustively discuss all available strategies. As such, we focus on illustrating two integrative strategies, not because they are necessarily the most widely used. Rather, these two integrative strategies and their usage assumptions descend from distinct theoretical traditions. One strategy descends from rater bias models, whereas the other strategy descends from social context models. Given the stark differences between rater bias and social context models, the two integrative strategies on which we focus provide ideal tests of the performance of competing approaches to integrating data produced by scholarship in youth development.

2.1 Trifactor Model

Rater bias models focus on how informant-specific factors (i.e., subjective bias) compromise the validity of reports (De Los Reyes & Epkins, 2023), with one influential model being the depression→distortion hypothesis (Richters, 1992). The depression→distortion hypothesis served as the conceptual foundation for the *Trifactor Model* (Bauer et al., 2013). Broadly, users of the Trifactor Model seek to remove variance unique to each informant's report to maximize common variance estimates. The Trifactor Model adheres to the notion that common variance among informants signals the "true" level of the domain being assessed. By logical extension, the Trifactor Model adheres to Compensating Operations, in that it treats discrepant results as measurement confounds.

The Trifactor Model includes three levels of latent factors. These factors each represent a source of variability contributing to individual informants' reports of a target's behavior, such as a child undergoing a clinical evaluation. First, the *Common Factor* is defined as the consensus among informants in the target's behavior being

B. A. Makol et al., *Youth Development in Context*, Springer Series on Child and Family Studies, https://doi.org/10.1007/978-3-031-80549-3_2

rated. Bauer et al. (2013) stated that this factor captures both the construct being assessed as well as shared sources of variability. These shared sources include similarities in informants' observational contexts (e.g., two teachers at school), similar roles of the informant relative to the target (e.g., two parents), or direct information sharing among informants (e.g., information provided at a parent-teacher conference). Second, *Perspective Factors* are defined as the unique views or biases of individual informants (e.g., parent depression) as well as other independent sources of variation that contribute to informants' ratings. These independent sources include informants' unique observational contexts (e.g., home vs. school) and roles relative to the target (e.g., parent vs. teacher). Thus, the Trifactor Model's *Perspective Factors* are theorized to capture information about unique views, biases, observational contexts, and roles. This suggests that *Perspective Factors* may capture both valid variations in informants' reports as well as measurement confounds in their reports. Yet, what this also means is that within *Perspective Factors*, users cannot distinguish variance reflecting valid data from variance reflecting measurement confounds. The lack of attention to isolating domain-relevant variance in *Perspective Factors* is consistent with the larger goal of the Trifactor Model. In fact, the developers of the Trifactor Model state this goal plainly in their 2013 paper, to "generate integrative scores that are purged of the subjective biases of single informants" (p. 475). Third, the Trifactor Model includes *Specific Factors*—item-level variations in informants' ratings. In theory, *Specific Factors* allow users to separate out informant-specific variance contributing to ratings at the item level, resulting in a refined estimate of the measured domain.

Bauer et al. (2013) developed two versions of the Trifactor Model (see Fig. 2.1). The *Unconditional Trifactor Model* includes the three latent variables that are conceptually defined and mathematically modeled by imposing constraints on factor loadings and factor correlations. First, all informant ratings are loaded onto the *Common Factor*, given that this factor represents the consensus view or shared variability in item responses across informants (i.e., common variance). Second, unique *Perspective Factors* are loaded onto each informants' ratings, which capture unique variance for each informant that is unshared with the other informants. Restrictions on model parameters can be imposed that allow researchers to model informants as *interchangeable* (i.e., randomly drawn from one set of raters) or *structurally different* (i.e., selected for the unique information provided; Eid et al., 2008). However, there is a lack of clarity on criteria for determining how to model informants (e.g., based on statistical tests of invariance or the extent to which informants are conceptually similar) across applications of the Trifactor Model (e.g., two parents are at times modeled as interchangeable and at other times are modeled as structurally different; Bauer et al., 2013; Haeny et al., 2018). Finally, *Specific Factors* are modeled to capture unique variance attributable to individual items in the model. Each factor in the Trifactor Model is assumed to be orthogonal to all other factors.

Bauer et al. (2013) also described a *Conditional Trifactor Model*, which extends the Unconditional Trifactor Model by including predictors of the factors in the model, including factors hypothesized to contribute to biases in informants' ratings. Specifically, one might include predictors of informants' ratings at the target level

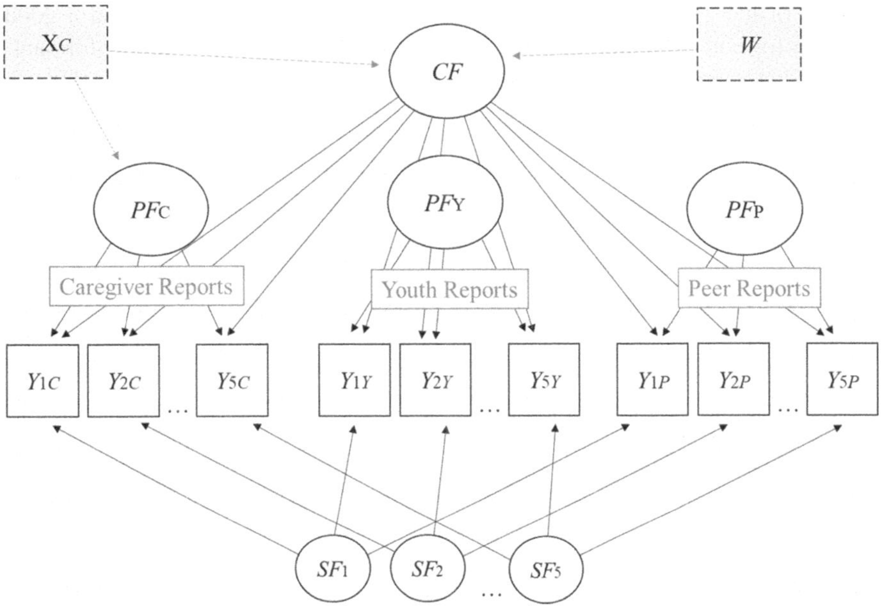

Fig. 2.1 Trifactor Model for parallel multi-informant reports on a five-item measure. Observed item ratings are numbered by item. *C*, *Y*, and *P* subscripts are for caregiver, youth, and peer confederate ratings, respectively. The *Common Factor* (*CF*), *Perspective Factors* (*PFs*), and *Specific Factors* (*SFs*) are modeled from observed item ratings. Dashed lines indicate additional model inputs in the Conditional Trifactor Model. Informant-specific predictors are denoted with an *X* and are loaded onto the relevant PF as well as the CF. Target-level predictors are denoted with a *W* and are loaded onto the CF. (Figure adapted from Bauer et al., 2013)

(e.g., youth gender) or informant level (e.g., parent depression). Bauer and colleagues argued that including predictors results in increased precision of score estimates, as this allows model users to test hypotheses about sources of variability contributing to informants' reports and remove variability thought to reflect informants' subjective biases. However, Bauer and colleagues did not provide guidance on how to use theory or empirical work to select predictors to include in the model.

2.1.1 Original Application of the Trifactor Model

In their original study, Bauer et al. (2013) applied their Trifactor Model to mother and father reports of youth negative affect using 13 parallel items from the Child Behavior Checklist (CBCL; Achenbach, 2001). The sample consisted of youth aged 2–18 years, with the sample split between youth who had a parent with substance use concerns and matched controls. The researchers included a *calibration sample*—a sample used to fit, evaluate, and refine the Trifactor Models being tested. The researchers also included a *cross-validation sample*—a sample used to evaluate the stability of the Trifactor Models being tested. Bauer et al. (2013) found a good model fit for both the Unconditional and Conditional Trifactor Models. Informant-level predictors included the mother's and father's lifetime history of an alcohol use disorder, depression or dysthymia, and antisocial personality disorder. The researchers did not include any measure of *current* parent mental health functioning. This is an important omission. With the Trifactor Model's foundation in the depression→distortion hypothesis, it logically follows that when evaluating rater biases, an informant's current functioning should factor into probing how they rate behavior, particularly when using items from the measure of current behavior the authors used in their study—the CBCL (i.e., youth behavior within the last 6 months; Achenbach, 2001). Parents with a lifetime history of dysthymia or depression and antisocial personality disorder were more likely to rate higher levels of child negative affect compared to parents without this lifetime history. The researchers concluded that these parents perceived their child's affect to be "greater than it is commonly perceived to be" (p. 486).

In effect, the Trifactor Model treats the *Common Factor* (i.e., an estimate of what informants commonly perceive) as the lone source of domain-relevant or valid variance. This is consistent with the aim of the Trifactor Model as stated by Bauer et al. (2013): to "generate integrative scores that are purged of the subjective biases of single informants" (p. 475). As such, the authors characterized unique variance estimates for parents' reports as measurement confounds. The Trifactor Model's "purging" of unique variance flows from its usage assumptions, a concept we first covered in Chap. 1. It also can have a profound effect on the criterion-related validity of scores taken from this model. As evidence of this, consider that Bauer and colleagues found that standardized factor loadings for the *Common Factor* were often lower than for the *Perspective Factors* and *Specific Factors*. Beyond usage assumptions, this observation compels us to return to another concept about which we learned in Chap. 1, namely, data conditions. Consistent with the usage assumptions of the Trifactor Model, the researchers interpreted this pattern of factor loadings as indicating that the "true" level of the domain being rated contributes less variance to informants' ratings than do informant- or item-level factors. Yet, if the data conditions to which a scholar applies the Trifactor Model violate the model's usage assumptions, then the scholar may incorrectly characterize sources of "true" or domain-relevant variance as measurement confounds. Under data conditions in which unique variance may contain valid data, the Trifactor Model places an artificial ceiling on the amount of valid data that scholars leverage to predict or explain domain-relevant phenomena.

The researchers conducted sensitivity analyses in which the final model was applied to the cross-validation sample and found an overall excellent fit when comparing intercepts, loadings, and factor regression parameter estimates. Bauer et al. (2013) also correlated the *Common Factor* with other integrative strategies including (a) the average proportion of items endorsed by parents, (b) the average proportion of items endorsed by either mothers or fathers, (c) the average factor score estimates obtained in a two-parameter logistic item response theory model, and (d) the average factor score estimates obtained in a moderated nonlinear factor analysis model. The researchers found that the *Common Factor* correlated at large magnitudes with all other integrative scores (*r*s = 0.79–0.84) but that the other integrative scores correlated with each other at even larger magnitudes (*r*s = 0.93–0.99). Bauer and colleagues concluded that although all integrative strategies assessed negative affect, the Trifactor Model produced a more interpretable score due to separating out unique sources of variance and removing variance thought to reflect parents' subjective biases. Yet the researchers did not evaluate the ability of the *Common Factor*, or other integrative scores, to predict independent criterion variables. Thus, the validity of data derived from the Trifactor Model (i.e., incremental, criterion-related), and in particular the *Common Factor*, awaits proper testing.

2.2 Concluding Comments

Taken together, although the Trifactor Model rests on a conceptual foundation (i.e., depression→distortion hypothesis), this foundation only informs modeling common variance. The Trifactor Model does not emphasize theory when making some important model-related decisions (e.g., selecting informants). Rather, the Trifactor Model compels its users to assume that all informants' reports inherently contain bias, and applying a factor analytic approach allows one to arrive at an integrative score that is "purged" of bias. Along these lines, those who implement the Trifactor Model must impose its usage assumptions at multiple steps of the modeling process. If the data conditions violate these usage assumptions, then it logically follows that model modifications must be made. For example, informants in the Trifactor Model can be modeled as structurally similar by imposing equal item intercepts and factor loadings for each informant. Thus, applying the Trifactor Model requires users to make numerous sample-specific modifications to yield an acceptable model fit. In this way, use of the Trifactor Model may result in over-specified models. This over-specification logically results in (a) decreased clarity when interpreting factors in the Trifactor Model for any one study, (b) increased uncertainty when comparing findings across Trifactor Model studies, and thus (c) barriers when seeking to understand the generalizability of findings for studies that use the Trifactor Model. As an integrative strategy, how does the Trifactor Model differ from an integrative strategy that descends from social context models? Chapter 3 addresses this question.

References

Achenbach, T. M. (2001). *Child behavior checklist for ages 6 to 18*. University of Vermont Research Center for Children, Youth, and Families.

Bauer, D. J., Howard, A. L., Baldasaro, R. E., Curran, P. J., Hussong, A. M., Chassin, L., & Zucker, R. A. (2013). A trifactor model for integrating ratings across multiple informants. *Psychological Methods, 18*(4), 475–493. https://psycnet.apa.org/doi/10.1037/a0032475

De Los Reyes, A., & Epkins, C. C. (2023). Introduction to the special issue. A dozen years of demonstrating that informant discrepancies are more than measurement error: Toward guidelines for integrating data from multi-informant assessments of youth mental health. *Journal of Clinical Child and Adolescent Psychology, 52*(1), 1–18. https://doi.org/10.1080/15374416.2022.2158843

Eid, M., Nussbeck, F. W., Geiser, C., Cole, D. A., Gollwitzer, M., & Lischetzke, T. (2008). Structural equation modeling of multitrait-multimethod data: Different models for different types of methods. *Psychological Methods, 13*(3), 230–253. https://doi.org/10.1037/a0013219

Haeny, A. M., Littlefield, A. K., Wood, P. K., & Sher, K. J. (2018). Method effects of the relation between family history of alcoholism and parent reports of offspring impulsive behavior. *Addictive Behaviors, 87*, 251–259. https://doi.org/10.1016/j.addbeh.2018.07.022

Richters, J. E. (1992). Depressed mothers as informants about their children: A critical review of the evidence for distortion. *Psychological Bulletin, 112*(3), 485–499. https://doi.org/10.1037/0033-2909.112.3.485

Chapter 3
Strategies for Integrating Behavioral Data: Social Context Models of Youth Development

In Chap. 2, we reviewed an integrative strategy informed by rater bias models. We learned about the assumptions underlying the use of the Trifactor Model—a strategy for integrating data that was informed by a widely used rater bias model, the depression→distortion hypothesis. In line with rater bias models, using the Trifactor Model requires making an assumption—that discrepant results cannot contain valid data. This assumption compels users to emphasize in their integrative strategy specific kinds of what we call *research practices*—in this case, consequential decisions about integrating data. Users of the Trifactor Model—or for that matter, any integrative strategy informed by rater bias models—engage in research practices that prioritize the precise estimation of common variance, which we covered in Chap. 1. However, these research practices compel users to deemphasize the precise estimation of unique variance, like what is captured in discrepant results. What if an integrative strategy tried to capture valid data in both common and unique variance? This chapter addresses this larger question. It presents an integrative strategy grounded in social context models, with assumptions and research practices that lie in stark contrast to those of rater bias models and, by extension, the Trifactor Model.

3.1 Satellite Model

Social context models focus on how discrepant results enhance measurement validity when assessing youth behavior (De Los Reyes & Epkins, 2023). As we learned in Chap. 1, one influential social context model is situational specificity (Achenbach et al., 1987). In the early 2000s, situational specificity served as the conceptual foundation for the *Satellite Model* (Kraemer et al., 2003). Key to the use of the Satellite Model is the strategic selection of structurally different informants, namely, those who vary in the contexts (e.g., home vs. school) and perspectives (e.g., self vs. other) from which they rate youth behavior (see Fig. 3.1). Stated another way, the

B. A. Makol et al., *Youth Development in Context*, Springer Series on Child and Family Studies, https://doi.org/10.1007/978-3-031-80549-3_3

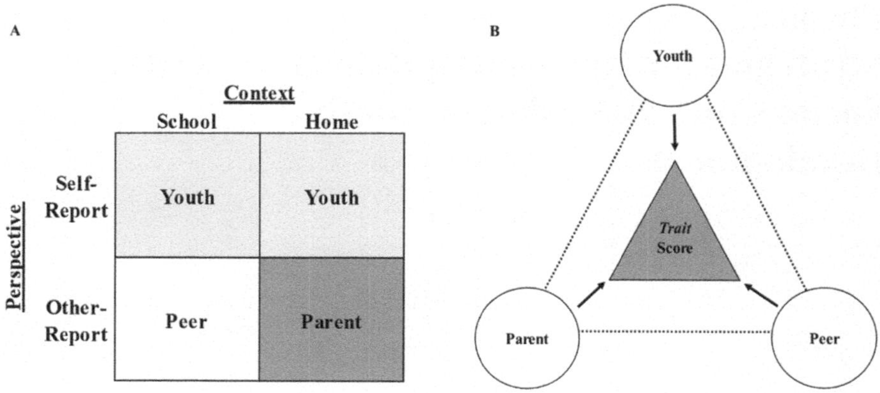

Fig. 3.1 Panel A depicts an example of the "mix-and-match" criterion to identify optimal informants to include in a multi-informant assessment. Informants systematically vary in the perspective and context from which they rate youth behavior, with the goal of effectively triangulating on a *Trait* score. Panel B provides a graphical depiction of multi-informant reports triangulating, much like the global positioning system, to identify the *Trait* score. Both peer and parent reports provide information from an other perspective, with peers providing information about the school context and parents providing information about the home context. Youth reports provide the self-perspective and information about both the school and home contexts. (Reproduced from the accepted manuscript version of Makol et al., 2020)

Satellite Model hinges on identifying factors (i.e., context and perspective) that produce domain-relevant discrepancies among structurally different informants' reports (Fig. 3.2) and thus require informants who vary within and between these factors.

The concepts underlying the Satellite Model are analogous to the global positioning systems used to track objects or people in geographic space. Global positioning systems acquire accurate location data from an array of satellites. The process of positioning satellites in the array focuses on placing each satellite at a strategically identified location, based on estimates of latitude and longitude. This process ensures that all satellites in the array lie in distinct points in space (Fig. 3.3, Panel A). These discrepancies in the positioning of satellites explain how global positioning systems produce accurate location estimates. Three satellites placed at the same latitude and longitude in geographic space make for a rather inaccurate system for locating an object. In contrast, three satellites placed at varying latitudes and longitudes—forming a *triangulated* position relative to the object's location—will, on average, optimize the accuracy of location information (Fig. 3.3, Panel B).

When applying the logic of global positioning systems to assessing behavior, Kraemer et al. (2003) argued for the importance of identifying factors that allow assessors to systematically "mix and match" the three informants used in the Satellite Model (see Fig. 3.1, Panel A). With global positioning systems, the goal is to triangulate satellite positions to estimate a target's location, using latitudes and longitudes to guide this positioning. When applied to behavior, treating informants like satellites should involve strategically varying their own "positioning" relative to

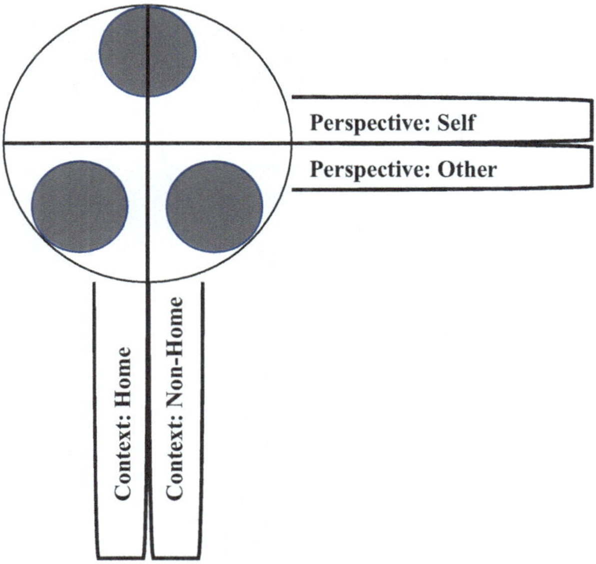

Fig. 3.2 Context and perspective as domain-relevant factors derived from the Satellite Model advanced by Kraemer et al. (2003). (Reproduced from the accepted manuscript version of De Los Reyes, 2024)

the other informants in the "satellite array." These variations should correspond to meaningful differences among the informants in how they observe and rate behavior. As such, the Satellite Model requires users to identify factors that validly predict or explain the discrepancies observed among informants' reports (Fig. 3.1, Panel B). When applied to behavior, the mixing and matching done within the assessment is a strategic task that involves selecting informants for whom theory and research indicate their reports will disagree and for valid reasons (Fig. 3.4). As stated by Kraemer and colleagues, "[T]he lack of correlation (orthogonality) between informants, to date considered problematic, becomes precisely the phenomenon that facilitates a more valid measure" (p. 1568). In this way, Kraemer and colleagues argued for an approach that markedly departs from that of Bauer and colleagues (2013). The unique variance reflected by discrepant results enhances the precision, accuracy, and thus criterion-related validity of multi-informant data. As such, the Satellite Model adheres to Converging and Diverging Operations, in that the use of the model involves hypothesizing domain-relevant sources of both common and unique variance when integrating multi-informant data.

To implement the Satellite Model, Kraemer et al. (2003) applied principal components analysis to multi-informant reports. This statistical approach linearly transforms a set of variables into a set of uncorrelated variables (Dunteman, 1989). Further, it is an exploratory technique that has no underlying statistical model. Rather, it reduces dimensionality among a set of variables to both enhance their interpretability and facilitate their use in subsequent analyses (e.g., as predictors and/or outcomes). The ingenuity of the Satellite Model, in large part, comes from

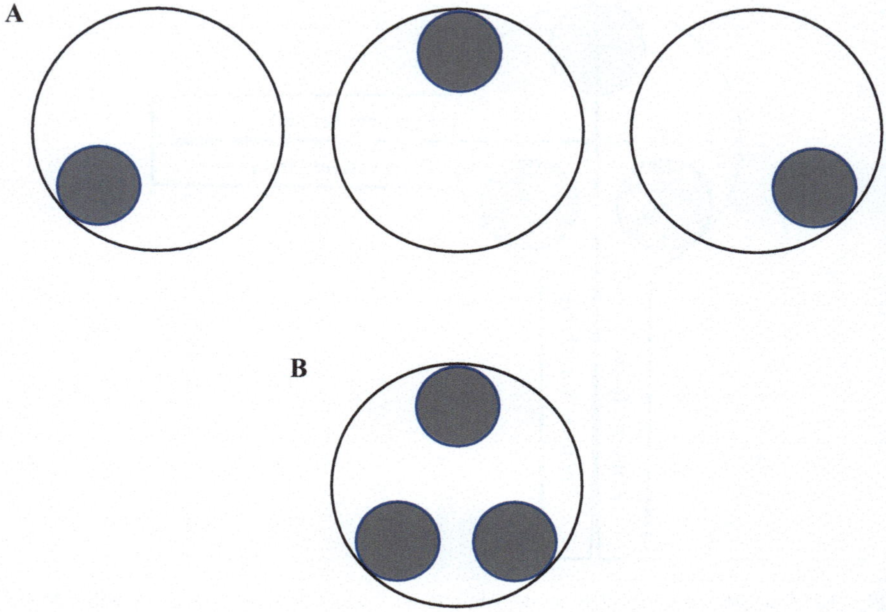

Fig. 3.3 Discrepant results in reports about behavior commonly reflect "moving targets" across the data sources used to assess behavioral domains (**a**). Thus, strategic selection of informants should translate into not only discrepant results that validly reflect the domains being assessed, but also, in combination with one another, explain far more variance in behavioral domains than approaches that assume that a single "bullseye" characterizes the only location where valid data can be found (**b**). Reproduced from the accepted manuscript version of De Los Reyes (2024)

the fact that it is more than an analytic technique. It fuses principal components analysis with a conceptually grounded approach to integrating informants' reports. For instance, the notion that the Satellite Model requires users to select informants whose reports will validly differ from each other compels users to strategically select structurally different informants to input into their models. The use of structurally different informants aligns with the modeling parameters and assumptions that underlie principal components analysis, as it yields linear composites of a set of latent variables, with each composite being orthogonal to all other composites. Further, the use of this approach involves carefully selecting theoretically meaningful items that are correlated but not redundant (Fabrigar & Wegener, 2011; Nunnally & Bernstein, 1994; Tabachnick & Fidell, 2013). In line with the use of principal components analysis, the Satellite Model requires a user to select structurally different informants who systematically vary in ways that result in low-to-moderate convergence among reports and with each informant contributing incrementally valid information when assessing youth behavior. Stated another way, the Satellite Model requires informants whose reports agree a little but validly disagree a lot.

When strategically selecting informants for use in a Satellite Model, Kraemer et al. (2003) argued that three component can be accurately identified through examination of component weights. Specifically, one component (i.e., *Trait* score)

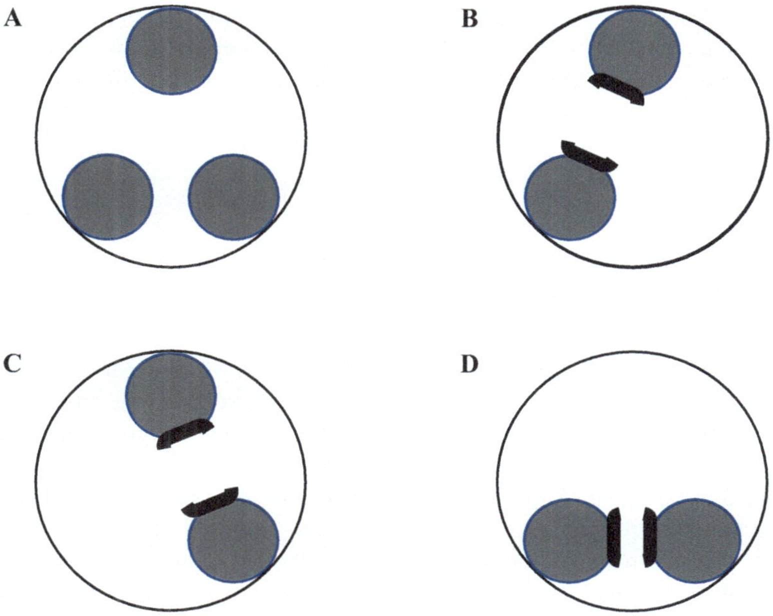

Fig. 3.4 Triangulation among data sources (**a**) and the discrepant results between structurally different data sources (**b**, **c**, and **d**). Note: The brackets in between data sources signal the presence of domain-relevant information in the discrepant results produced between sources. (Reproduced from the accepted manuscript version of De Los Reyes, 2024)

reflects variability for which all three informants' reports load strongly and in the same direction (e.g., all three informants' reports display loadings ≥0.40). As the first component obtained in a principal component analysis, the *Trait* score explains the most variance in informants' reports and is the key integrative score to be used in subsequent analyses. A second component (i.e., *Context* score) reflects informants' contexts such that informants from different contexts load in opposite directions (e.g., parents have positive loadings vs. teachers have negative loadings). A third component (i.e., *Perspective* score) reflects informants' perspectives such that self-reports load in the opposite direction of observer informants' reports (e.g., youths have positive loadings vs. parents/teachers have negative loadings). In this respect, inspecting component weights allows users to "check" whether the informants they selected produced variations that conform to expectations. Beyond these components, Kraemer and colleagues stated that their model allows for error or random factors related to the assessment process but conceptualizes this error as explaining only a small, insignificant amount of variance in informants' reports. Importantly, this allowance of error is normally a key problem in the use of factor analytic techniques, particularly when using items of uncertain psychometric value (e.g., individual item responses; Nunnally & Bernstein, 1994). However, researchers typically apply the Satellite Model to examining not individual items, but rather summary scores taken from informants' reports on well-established instruments.

Further, as mentioned previously, much of the literature on discrepant results focuses on informants' reports based on the use of thoroughly studied instrumentation (see Achenbach, 2020; De Los Reyes & Epkins, 2023). Thus, because Satellite Model users select instruments capable of producing discrepant results that contain valid data, they can have a fair degree of certainty as to the outcomes of the data analytic models that they construct.

3.1.1 Original Application of the Satellite Model

In their original study, Kraemer et al. (2003) applied the Satellite Model to mother, teacher, and child reports of internalizing problems, externalizing problems, and academic functioning. Mothers and teachers completed parallel forms of the MacArthur Health and Behavior Questionnaire (Essex et al., 2001), and children completed the Berkeley Puppet Interview (Ablow et al., 1999). Kraemer and colleagues observed that for each area of functioning assessed, these reports, which met the "mix-and-match criterion" graphically depicted in Fig. 3.1, yielded component weights consistent with *Trait* (i.e., all informants' reports loaded strongly and in the same direction), *Context* (i.e., mother reports loaded in the opposite direction of teacher reports, with child reports loading between mother and teacher reports), and *Perspective* scores (i.e., self-reports loaded in the opposite direction of mother and teacher reports). Interestingly, Kraemer and colleagues also applied the Satellite Model to three informants who did not meet their mix-and-match criterion. Specifically, using the same sample, the researchers applied the Satellite Model to mother, father, and teacher reports of internalizing problems. When doing so, they found that principal component analysis did not yield component weights consistent with *Trait*, *Context*, or *Perspective* scores. Thus, implementing the Satellite Model requires a strategic selection of informants whose reports "fit" assumptions underlying its use. If a user enters informants into the model whose reports do not systematically vary along key dimensions, then the component scores will fail to yield expected component weights. The Satellite Model harbors falsifiability in model testing that adheres to social context models of discrepant results.

Kraemer et al.'s (2003) original Satellite Model study did not include validation tests of scores derived from the model. Nearly 20 years later, Makol et al. (2020) conducted exactly these validation tests. Specifically, they applied the Satellite Model to caregiver and adolescent reports of adolescent social anxiety, along with a third informant (i.e., *peer confederate*) who interacted with adolescents within a laboratory-controlled set of tasks designed to simulate how adolescents interact with same-age unfamiliar peers (Fig. 3.5). These informants systematically varied in the context (i.e., home vs. non-home context) and perspective (i.e., self vs. other) from which they observed adolescent social anxiety. Consistent with the development of the Satellite Model, Makol and colleagues found that the *Trait* score demonstrated incremental validity in two ways. First, the *Trait* score predicted adolescent referral status (i.e., community control vs. clinical-referred group; odds ratios

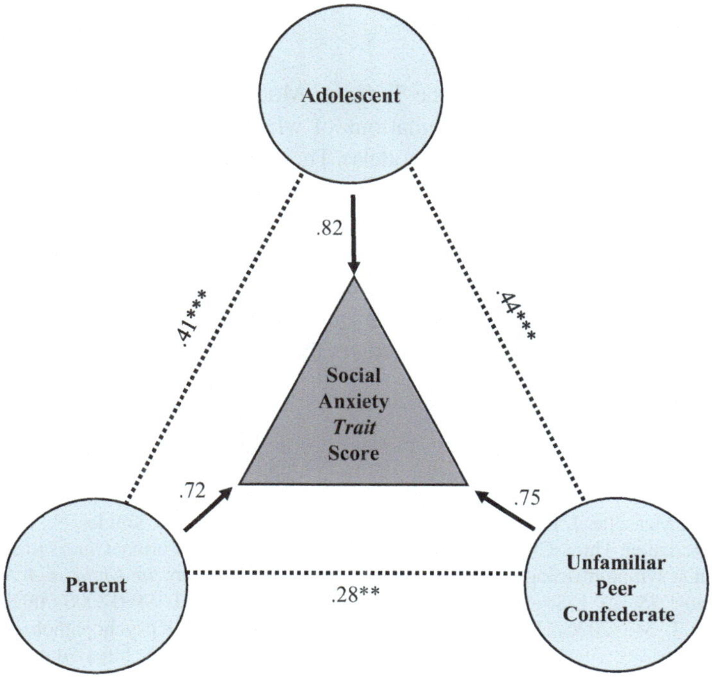

Fig. 3.5 Graphical depiction of multiple informants' reports triangulating in an application of Kraemer et al.'s (2003) Satellite Model. Note: Values on dotted lines denote bivariate correlations among parent, adolescent, and peer confederate reports of adolescent social anxiety. Values on solid arrows denote component weights from principal component analysis of parent, adolescent, and peer confederate reports. $^{**}p < 0.01$; $^{***}p < 0.001$. (Reproduced from the accepted manuscript version of Makol et al., 2020)

[ORs] = 2.66–6.53), over-and-above individual informants' reports. Second, the *Trait* score predicted ratings from trained independent observers of the levels of social anxiety that the adolescent displayed when interacting with peer confederates (i.e., βs = 0.47–0.67), again over-and-above individual informants' reports. Taken together, Makol and colleagues applied the Satellite Model to a set of data conditions in which the criterion-related validity evidence supported its usage assumptions.

Kraemer et al.'s (2003) Satellite Model has some limitations. First, it is designed to be used with three or more informants and may not be suitable for assessments leveraging only two informants. Further, determining whether one has appropriately identified the components is a qualitative process (i.e., examining component weights for "Trait," "Context," "Perspective") and one for which Kraemer and colleagues do not offer thresholds. Finally, principal components analysis is an exploratory technique, making it inappropriate to use as a hypothesis testing tool when interpreting factor structures (Tabachnick & Fidell, 2013). As such, when using the Satellite Model, it is imperative to leverage validation testing strategies to gauge the validity of interpreting observed components (see also Charamut et al., 2022).

3.2 Concluding Comments

Chapters 2 and 3 described how the Trifactor Model and the Satellite Model each stem from distinct theoretical foundations of what discrepant results reflect (i.e., rater bias models vs. social context models). These theoretical foundations place the Trifactor Model and the Satellite Model on diverse paths in terms of analytic modeling and, by extension, the process of integrating multi-informant data. As such, if the theoretical foundations point toward distinct sources of variance regarding discrepant results, then what are the implications for how researchers implement the models? In Chap. 4, we probe this larger question inspired by Chaps. 2 and 3 in a way that sets the foundation for the chapters that follow.

References

Ablow, J. C., Measelle, J. R., Kraemer, H. C., Harrington, R., Luby, J., Smider, N., et al. (1999). The MacArthur Three-City outcome study: Evaluating multi-informant measures of young children's symptomatology. *Journal of the American Academy of Child and Adolescent Psychiatry, 38*(12), 1580–1590. https://doi.org/10.1097/00004583-199912000-00020

Achenbach, T. M. (2020). Bottom-up and top-down paradigms for psychopathology: A half-century odyssey. *Annual Review of Clinical Psychology, 16*, 1–24. https://doi.org/10.1146/annurev-clinpsy-071119-115831

Achenbach, T. M., McConaughy, S. H., & Howell, C. T. (1987). Child/adolescent behavioral and emotional problems: Implications of cross-informant correlations for situational specificity. *Psychological Bulletin, 101*(2), 213–232. https://psycnet.apa.org/doi/10.1037/0033-2909.101.2.213

Charamut, N. R., Racz, S. J., Wang, M., & De Los Reyes, A. (2022). Integrating multi-informant reports of youth mental health: A construct validation test of Kraemer and colleagues' (2003) Satellite Model. *Frontiers in Psychology, 13*, 911629. https://doi.org/10.3389/fpsyg.2022.911629

De Los Reyes, A. (2024). *Discrepant results in mental health research: What they mean, why they matter, and how they inform scientific practices*. Oxford University Press.

De Los Reyes, A., & Epkins, C. C. (2023). Introduction to the special issue. A dozen years of demonstrating that informant discrepancies are more than measurement error: Toward guidelines for integrating data from multi-informant assessments of youth mental health. *Journal of Clinical Child and Adolescent Psychology, 52*(1), 1–18. https://doi.org/10.1080/15374416.2022.2158843

Dunteman, G. H. (1989). *Principal components analysis*. (No. 69. Sage.

Essex, M. J., Klein, M. H., Miech, R., & Smider, N. A. (2001). Timing of initial exposure to maternal major depression and children's mental health symptoms in kindergarten. *The British Journal of Psychiatry, 179*(2), 151–156. https://psycnet.apa.org/doi/10.1192/bjp.179.2.151

Fabrigar, L. R., & Wegener, D. T. (2011). *Exploratory factor analysis*. Oxford University Press.

Kraemer, H. C., Measelle, J. R., Ablow, J. C., Essex, M. J., Boyce, W. T., & Kupfer, D. J. (2003). A new approach to integrating data from multiple informants in psychiatric assessment and research: Mixing and matching contexts and perspectives. *American Journal of Psychiatry, 160*(9), 1566–1577. https://doi.org/10.1176/appi.ajp.160.9.1566

Makol, B. A., Youngstrom, E. A., Racz, S. J., Qasmieh, N., Glenn, L. E., & De Los Reyes, A. (2020). Integrating multiple informants' reports: How conceptual and measurement models may address long-standing problems in clinical decision-making. *Clinical Psychological Science, 8*(6), 953–970. https://doi.org/10.1177/2167702620924439

Nunnally, J. C., & Bernstein, I. H. (1994). *Psychometric theory* (3rd ed.). McGraw-Hill.

Tabachnick, B. G., & Fidell, L. S. (2013). *Using multivariate statistics* (6th ed.). Pearson.

Chapter 4
Strategies for Integrating Behavioral Data: Research Practices in Youth Development

Thus far, we have discussed how the Satellite Model and Trifactor Model differ in modeling approaches. We have also discussed how these approaches stem, in part, from the different conceptual foundations informing each of these models. Yet our discussions beg a key question: When scholars implement these integrative strategies, do they vary in their research practices? For example, do scholars using the Satellite Model differ from scholars using the Trifactor Model on which informants' reports they input into their analytic models? Do these strategies distinguish researchers in terms of how many informants' reports they input into their analytic models? This chapter probes these questions surrounding research practices. We first delve deeper into CONTEXT, which we first learned about in Chap. 1. CONTEXT grounds the studies we report in this book. To support this notion, we discuss the findings of meta-analytic work on scholars' use of the Satellite Model and Trifactor Model and how scholars vary in their research practices when implementing these integrative strategies. These two aims of this chapter set the stage for the two studies reported in this book, which we cover in Chaps. 5, 6, and 7.

4.1 CONTEXT, Research Practices, and Discrepant Results

As a measurement validation paradigm, CONTEXT also provides users with a theoretical foundation for how concepts surrounding discrepant results, along with philosophical stances on scientific inquiry generally, portend variations among scholars in their research practices when confronted with discrepant results. Understanding this foundation requires not only articulating the usage assumptions of CONTEXT, but also distinguishing them from those that underlie the validation paradigm that has historically guided measurement in youth development. To this end, we begin this conceptual discussion by delineating this traditional paradigm. Following this, we highlight key conceptual and epistemological differences between this

B. A. Makol et al., *Youth Development in Context*, Springer Series on Child and Family Studies, https://doi.org/10.1007/978-3-031-80549-3_4

traditional paradigm and CONTEXT, their links to the Satellite Model and Trifactor Model, and how these links reveal the ways in which users of integrative strategies vary in their research practices.

4.1.1 Multi-Trait-Multi-Method Matrix

To understand the validation paradigm that has historically dominated scholarship in measurement, we must first consider its own origins. In the mid-1950s, Garner and colleagues (1956) advanced the concept of Converging Operations, which we first learned about in Chap. 1 (Fig. 1.4, Panel A). It turns out that Converging Operations inspired the usage assumptions of this paradigm (Grace, 2001; Highhouse, 2009)—the *Multi-Trait-Multi-Method Matrix* (*MTMM*; Campbell & Fiske, 1959). The MTMM holds that strong evidence of score validity comes from observing high-magnitude correlations between scores taken from instruments that measure the same domains. Further, the greater the distinction or independence between the instruments' modalities (e.g., survey vs. behavioral observation), the greater the evidence supporting score validity (Fiske & Campbell, 1992). For these usage assumptions to make logical sense, the reverse must also be true. Low-magnitude correlations between scores taken from instruments that measure the same domains must signal weak evidence of score validity. Stated another way, when two instruments that measure the same domain produce scores that correlate weakly with each other, this must be the byproduct of factors that are irrelevant to whatever domain the instruments measure (i.e., measurement confounds). The MTMM fits data conditions for which these assumptions hold, but what happens when the data conditions violate these assumptions?

4.1.2 CONTEXT

As a validation paradigm, CONTEXT fits the very data conditions that violate the usage assumptions of the MTMM. CONTEXT is particularly well suited to guide measurement validation work in youth development—an area of scholarly work for which studies (a) produce discrepant results that (b) may contain domain-relevant information. In five major ways, CONTEXT guides scholarship on measurement down fundamentally distinct paths, relative to the guidance provided by the MTMM. We describe the first of these guides in Table 4.1, namely, theory. First, if users of the MTMM must assume that discrepant results can only reflect measurement confounds, then observing discrepant results should compel users to make hypotheses about the kinds of measurement confounds that these discrepancies reflect. In this respect, one can readily see the connection between the MTMM and the depression→distortion hypothesis. In contrast, users of CONTEXT seek to design studies premised on the notion that discrepant results might contain

Table 4.1 Differences between CONTEXT and the MTMM paradigm in guidance on theory surrounding discrepant results

Validation paradigm	Core assumption regarding discrepant results	How assumption guides conceptual foundations of paradigm-informed research	Examples of theories applied in prior research	Citations of prior work that applied paradigm-informed theories
MTMM	All discrepant results reflect measurement confounds	Guides users to apply theories about discrepant results that posit factors that produce rater biases	Depression-distortion hypothesis (Richters, 1992)	Bauer et al. (2013); Clark et al. (2016); Jungersen and Lonigan (2021); Olino et al. (2018); Olino et al. (2021)
CONTEXT	At least some discrepant results contain domain-relevant information	Guides users to apply theories about discrepant results that posit factors that produce domain-relevant information	Situational specificity (Achenbach et al., 1987)	De Los Reyes et al. (2022a, b, c); Deros et al. (2018); Lerner et al. (2017); Makol et al. (2020); Watts et al. (2022)

Note: Reproduced from the accepted manuscript version of De Los Reyes, Wang, et al. (2023a); *CONTEXT* Classifying Observations Necessitates Theory, Epistemology, and Testing, *MTMM* Multi-Trait Multi-Method Matrix

domain-relevant information. As such, they are most likely to turn to concepts such as situational specificity to guide their work.

Beyond theory, consider how users of these validation paradigms approach their work from the perspective of *Epistemology*—the branch of Philosophy focused on what is known and knowable (see Hempel, 1966). As seen in Table 4.2, if users of the MTMM assume that discrepant results reflect measurement confounds, then this assumption logically results in scholars discounting the possibility that discrepant results even count as "evidence." Consequently, they frequently develop ad hoc hypotheses for what these discrepancies represent, to preserve the veracity of the notion that common variance is the only source of valid data (e.g., discrepant results must reflect measurement confounds). Importantly, these ad hoc hypotheses have a core feature—they cannot be falsified. Users of the MTMM do not follow up with empirical tests that scrutinize whether their ad hoc hypothesis accurately characterizes the discrepancies they observed (see also De Los Reyes, Wang, et al., 2023a). In contrast, CONTEXT guides users to construct studies that directly test the hypothesis that discrepant results contain valid data. As such, these tests encourage users to follow up on null findings regarding the hypothesis. Consider a user whose initial tests produced inconclusive findings that the discrepant results produced by their assessments contain domain-relevant data. Under these circumstances, CONTEXT compels users to construct subsequent tests of whether the discrepant results they observe are accurately characterized as measurement confounds. Unlike the MTMM, CONTEXT guides users to take a hypothesis-driven and empirically based approach to probing what discrepant results reflect.

Table 4.2 Differences between CONTEXT and the MTMM paradigm in epistemology surrounding discrepant results

Validation paradigm	Test implication	Logical extension of test implication	Research practices that logically extend from test implication	Relevant citations
MTMM	Converging findings are the only data to contain domain-relevant information	Anything less than converging findings ought to be interpreted as inconclusive evidence	Primary outcome measure methods; tests of measurement invariance; use of structural models that prioritize common variance; eschew estimating common or unique variance altogether and just examine informants' reports individually	Bauer et al. (2013); Boutron et al. (2010); De Los Reyes et al. (2011); Howe et al. (2019); Olino et al. (2018)
CONTEXT	At least some discrepant results reflect domain-relevant information	Discrepant results may optimize rather than hinder the interpretability of findings	Strategic selection of informants that produce context-sensitive information; use of analytic strategies that facilitate identifying discrepant results and testing whether they contain domain-relevant information	Deros et al. (2018); Kraemer et al. (2003); Laird (2020); Lakind et al. (2022); Makol et al. (2020)

Note: Reproduced from the accepted manuscript version of De Los Reyes et al. (2023a); *CONTEXT* Classifying Observations Necessitates Theory, Epistemology, and Testing, *MTMM* Multi-Trait Multi-Method Matrix

The combination of theoretical and epistemological distinctions between CONTEXT and the MTMM logically leads users of these validation paradigms down distinct paths in terms of their research practices when working with multi-informant data. Put simply, if users of the MTMM assume that discrepant results reflect measurement confounds, then the informants themselves can be nothing more than the means through which they can obtain sound estimates of common variance (Table 4.3). We first learned about common variance in Chap. 1. In Chap. 2, we learned that in formative demonstrations of the Trifactor Model (Bauer et al., 2013), the developers tested its fit with informants who tend to provide reports that are highly correlated (e.g., reports from two or more caregivers; see De Los Reyes et al., 2015). If these informants are the means through which users of the MTMM observe high degrees of common variance, then any of the informants' domain-relevant characteristics (e.g., the structural differences between informants and where they observe behavior) are of little importance. In contrast, CONTEXT guides users to select informants precisely because of the structural differences between their reports. This is because CONTEXT guides users to detect valid data in multiple informants' reports and by using sources of data beyond informants' responses to the instruments they complete. CONTEXT guides users to detect valid

Table 4.3 Differences between CONTEXT and the MTMM paradigm in guidance on research practices surrounding the selection of informants

Validation paradigm	Central focus of paradigm	Treatment of individual informants' reports that logically result from focus	Research practice that logically extends from focus	Relevant citations
MTMM	Attain precise estimates of common variance	If the means for selecting informants is to achieve the end of estimating common variance, then no one informant's report has value unique to itself; each report simply reflects an "error" around a measure of central tendency (i.e., common variance)	Select multiple informants for the sole purpose of maximizing precision in estimating common variance; the actual informants do not matter (e.g., could be structurally different, random raters, parents, teachers, youth, peers), so long as one attains precise estimates of common variance	Bauer et al. (2013); Edgeworth (1888); Fiske and Campbell (1992); Roberts and Caspi (2001)
CONTEXT	Strike a balance between attaining precise estimates of both common variance and domain-relevant unique variance (i.e., discrepant results)	If the means of the multi-informant approach involve collecting reports from structurally different informants and the discrepant results produced with this approach ought to contain domain-relevant information, then determining which specific informants will provide reports is as an important decision as determining the content of the measures the informants will complete	Strategically select informants who will produce both common variance and discrepant results that contain domain-relevant information; the actual informants are instrumental in optimizing measurement validity	De Los Reyes et al. (2009); Kraemer et al. (2003); Makol et al. (2020)

Note: Reproduced from the accepted manuscript version of De Los Reyes et al. (2023a); *CONTEXT* Classifying Observations Necessitates Theory, Epistemology, and Testing, *MTMM* Multi-Trait Multi-Method Matrix

data using the structural differences between informants. In line with the notion of situational specificity, this typically comes in the form of examining whether discrepant results reflect variations among informants in the social contexts in which they observe behavior (e.g., parent at home vs. teacher at school). Along these lines, we learned in Chap. 3 that the Satellite Model guides users to strategically select informants based on their structural differences (i.e., contexts and perspectives through which they observe the youth they rate; Kraemer et al., 2003).

Table 4.4 Differences between CONTEXT and the MTMM paradigm in guidance on research practices surrounding the selection of analytic strategies

Validation paradigm	Central focus of paradigm	Logical result of focus	Research practices that logically extend from focus	Relevant citations
MTMM	Attain precise estimates of common variance, because discrepant results reflect measurement confounds	If discrepant results reflect measurement confounds, then there is no legitimate reason for modeling them, other than creating estimates of error for modeling purposes	Use of analytic strategies that cannot estimate the incremental value of discrepant results	Alvarez et al. (2021); Murray et al. (2021); Olino et al. (2018); Russell et al. (2016); van der Ende et al. (2020)
CONTEXT	Strike a balance between attaining precise estimates of both common variance and unique variance, because discrepant results may reflect domain-relevant information	If discrepant results may reflect domain-relevant information and common variance estimates are likely domain-relevant as well, then one must leverage analytic strategies that allow one to determine the relative value of both common and unique variance for the purpose of scholarly inquiry (e.g., characterizing behavior, predicting outcomes, theory testing)	Use of analytic strategies that facilitate testing for the incremental value of discrepant results	Becker-Haimes et al. (2018); De Los Reyes et al. (2009); Laird and De Los Reyes (2013); Makol et al. (2019); Makol et al. (2020)

Note: Reproduced from the accepted manuscript version of De Los Reyes et al. (2023a); *CONTEXT* Classifying Observations Necessitates Theory, Epistemology, and Testing, *MTMM* Multi-Trait Multi-Method Matrix

Given the theoretical distinctions between CONTEXT and the MTMM, it should be no surprise that the two validation paradigms vary in the guidance they provide users when selecting analytic strategies. Consider the process of selecting strategies for integrating data (Table 4.4). How well equipped would users of the MTMM be to select analytic strategies for integrating multi-informant data? Multi-informant assessments of youth behavior commonly produce highly discrepant results. A user of the MTMM cannot rely on this paradigm to detect valid data in a source of variance that the paradigm assumes only reflects measurement confounds. Thus, the MTMM guides users to assume that discrepancies reflect measurement confounds and that means users select analytic strategies that are geared toward modeling common variance. As we and others have noted (e.g., De Los Reyes et al., 2023a, b; Howe et al., 2019), these procedures then focus their attention on a small amount of valid data to understand or explain youth behavior. In contrast to the MTMM, CONTEXT guides users to select analytic strategies that are capable of modeling valid data from multiple sources (i.e., common and unique variance), not just one. The Satellite Model represents one of these strategies, but it is not the only strategy available (for a review, see De Los Reyes, 2024).

If CONTEXT and the MTMM vary in research practices surrounding the selection of informants and analytic strategies, then it would be reasonable to distinguish these paradigms as to the guidance they provide users when designing validation studies. We summarize these differences in Table 4.5. An important distinction between these two paradigms stems from how the MTMM's assumptions about discrepant results extend to comparing scores taken from instruments constructed with distinct modalities. Users of the MTMM assume that discrepancies of all kinds reflect measurement confounds. This goes for discrepancies observed when informants produce scores on parallel versions of the same instrument (e.g., survey or interview; De Los Reyes et al., 2023a). This also goes for discrepancies observed when scores from instruments constructed with different modalities produce discrepant results (e.g., interview vs. performance-based task; De Los Reyes et al., 2019a, b). What this means is that, from a study design standpoint, users of the MTMM are ill-equipped to leverage variations among instruments to identify sources of valid data other than responses to the instruments themselves. In contrast, CONTEXT guides users to strategically select validity criteria that allow them to verify whether the discrepant results produced by informants contain valid data. Typically, these validity criteria contain structural characteristics of their own, in that they often reference behaviors that youth exhibit within specific contexts, including naturalistic observations of their behavior at school (e.g., De Los Reyes et al., 2022c), controlled observations of their behavior at home (e.g., De Los Reyes et al., 2009), and controlled observations of their behavior when interacting with peers (e.g., Makol et al., 2020). In each of these circumstances and many others (for a review, see De Los Reyes & Epkins, 2023), scholars have adopted CONTEXT-informed approaches to measurement validation that leverage the structural characteristics of independent validity criteria to detect valid data in discrepant results.

4.1.3 How Might Users of the MTMM and CONTEXT Vary in Their Research Practices?

Taken together, the MTMM and CONTEXT differ in fundamental ways in terms of how they conceptualize, model, and test competing ideas about discrepant results and the data they contain. These distinctions between MTMM and CONTEXT provide us with testable hypotheses about how users of these validation paradigms might approach even the most basic decisions regarding the use of multi-informant approaches to assessing youth behavior.

Table 4.5 Differences between CONTEXT and the MTMM paradigm in guidance on research practices surrounding study design

Validation paradigm	Core assumption regarding discrepant results	Logical result of focus	Research practices that logically extend from focus	Relevant citations
MTMM	All discrepant results reflect measurement confounds	If discrepant results reflect measurement confounds, then it is logical to assume that discrepancies between informants' reports, and other non-informant modalities (e.g., observed behavior) also reflect measurement confounds	Use of study designs that cannot distinguish discrepant results that reflect measurement confounds from those that reflect domain-relevant information	Bauer et al. (2013); De Los Reyes, Lerner, et al. (2019b); Dunning et al. (2004); van der Ende et al. (2020); Watts et al. (2022)
CONTEXT	At least some discrepant results contain unique domain-relevant information	If the means of the multi-informant approach involve collecting reports from structurally different informants and the discrepant results produced with this approach ought to contain domain-relevant information, then detecting this information requires careful attention to selecting non-informant modalities to serve as domain-relevant validity indicators; selecting validity indicators is as an important decision as selecting the informants	Use of study designs that facilitate distinguishing discrepant results that reflect measurement confounds from those that reflect domain-relevant information; these designs involve "matching" the structural characteristics of the informants providing reports with the structural characteristics of the non-informant modalities used to construct validity indicators	Al Ghriwati et al. (2018); De Los Reyes et al. (2009); De Los Reyes et al. (2013); De Los Reyes, Cook, et al. (2022c); Makol et al. (2019); Makol et al. (2020)

Note: Reproduced from the accepted manuscript version of De Los Reyes et al. (2023a); *CONTEXT* Classifying Observations Necessitates Theory, Epistemology, and Testing, *MTMM* Multi-Trait Multi-Method Matrix

Our overview of CONTEXT and how we can differentiate its core tenets from those of the MTMM provides a foundation for thinking about research practices when using the Satellite Model and Trifactor Model. This is because, whereas the Satellite Model's usage assumptions align more so with CONTEXT than the

MTMM, the Trifactor Model's usage assumptions align more so with the MTMM than CONTEXT. CONTEXT reveals a notion—that differences in the conceptual and epistemological foundations of these two integrative strategies portend that users of these strategies vary in how they make even the most basic decisions surrounding research practices. These decisions include how many informants users include in their models and whether the informants selected structurally vary from each other. Makol (2022) tested this notion in a systematic review of 47 studies.

4.2 Systematic Review of Research Practices Linked to Integrative Strategies

Makol (2022) probed studies that used the Trifactor Model or Satellite Model to integrate multi-informant data. A team of trained raters reliably coded studies on the number of informants. Coders also categorized informants by the kinds of contexts in which they observe youth, including the home context (i.e., mothers, fathers, caregivers), school context (i.e., teachers), peer context (i.e., peers), mixed contexts (i.e., self-reporters, clinicians), or various informants (i.e., multiple informant types combined, official records).

In Table 4.6, we report a subset of the larger study set on these key characteristics. Consistent with the data reported in Table 4.6, Makol (2022) found that Trifactor Model studies included informants representing two or greater contexts 50% of the time, whereas, the other 50% of the time, these studies included only mothers and fathers as the informants in the assessment (i.e., representing the home context only). Given our review of the Trifactor Model in Chap. 2, these research practices make sense. In fact, the informants used by Bauer et al. (2013) in their description of the Trifactor Model only included mothers and fathers—informants who tend to observe behavior in one context (i.e., home). Consequently, it would be natural to assume that if the illustration of the Trifactor Model by its developers (a) only used two informants who (b) collectively only observed behavior in a single context, then (c) it should be "acceptable" to implement this integrative strategy using the same kinds of informants.

In contrast to the use of the Trifactor Model, Satellite Model studies included informants representing two or greater contexts 90.7% of the time, with the most common application being consistent with Kraemer et al.'s (2003) original use of caregiver, youth, and teacher reports (60.5% of unique Satellite Model applications). Here as well, our review of the Satellite Model in Chap. 3 facilitates interpreting these findings. Unlike Bauer et al. (2013), Kraemer et al. provided users with explicit guidance on which kinds of informants to select and based in part on the contexts in which informants observe behavior. By extension, this guidance also informs the minimum number of informants' reports to integrate. In these respects, users of the Satellite Model do not have to "follow the lead" of the practices implemented by its developers in terms of which informants to input into their analytic

Table 4.6 Illustrative examples of Trifactor Model and Satellite Model studies

Study	Sample size	Developmental period	Construct measured	Number of informants	Informant context			
					Ho	Sc	Mix	Pr
Trifactor Model studies								
Bauer et al. (2013)	626	Early childhood, childhood, adolescence	Negative affect	2	✓^{m} ✓^{f}			
Chen et al. (2015)*	1132	Adulthood	Sexual openness	1			✓^{s}	
Clark et al. (2017)	273	Early childhood, childhood	Temperament	2	✓^{m} ✓^{f}			
Curran et al. (2020)	359	Adulthood	Depressive symptoms	2			✓^{s}	✓^{p}
Satellite Model studies								
Armstrong et al. (2014)	396	Childhood	Internalizing problems, externalizing problems	3	✓^{m}	✓^{t}	✓^{s}	
Gardner et al. (2008)	803	Adolescence, adulthood	Self-regulation, deviant peer affiliation	3	✓^{m}	✓^{t}	✓^{s}	
Kraemer et al. (2003)	539	Childhood	Emotional/ behavioral difficulties, academic problems	3	✓^{m}	✓^{t}	✓^{s}	
Owens and Hinshaw (2016)	140	Childhood, adolescence	Internalizing problems, externalizing problems	3	✓^{c}	✓^{t}	✓^{s}	

Note: Characteristics reported in this table were derived from data reported in Makol (2022) and based on the codes of trained, independent raters. Early childhood = 0–4 years; childhood = 5–12 years; adolescence = 13–18 years; adulthood = 18 or older; Ho = home; Sc = school; Pr = peer; ✓^{m} = mother; ✓^{f} = father; ✓^{t} = teacher; ✓^{p} = peer; ✓^{c} = caregiver; ✓^{s} = self. *In this study, four *Perspective Factors* were included, but all came from self-report

models and how many to input. Rather, built into the Satellite Model is a framework for conceptualizing the discrepant results produced by structurally different informants. This framework—rather than the developers' own research practices—guides the implementation of this integrative strategy. In fact, in Chap. 4, we describe a study that applied the Satellite Model with a fundamentally distinct set of informants than those used by its developers to illustrate its use. Given these key distinctions between the Trifactor Model and Satellite Model, it should come as no surprise that Makol (2022) found studies included significantly greater numbers of informants when applying the Satellite Model, relative to the number of informants used in studies that applied the Trifactor Model.

4.3 Concluding Comments

Taken together, Makol (2022) found that users of the Satellite Model input more informants into their models—and are more likely to include structurally different informants—relative to users of the Trifactor Model. Yet, as a systematic review, Makol did not address the implications of these research practices for how researchers apply these integrative strategies and the validity of the scores these strategies ultimately produce. These limitations of the Makol review take us back to key issues we raised in Chap. 1.

In Chap. 1, recall our discussion of data conditions—core characteristics of the scores taken from multi-informant assessments of youth behavior. Depending on the data conditions, the Trifactor Model may outperform the Satellite Model in terms of the validity of scores produced by the strategy, or vice versa. Importantly, Chaps. 2 and 3 revealed stark differences between the Trifactor Model and Satellite Model in terms of their usage assumptions, particularly regarding what discrepant results reflect and the sources of domain-relevant or valid data (i.e., only common variance vs. both common and unique variance). In fact, the differences in these strategies' assumptions stem in large part from their distinct theoretical foundations (i.e., depression→distortion hypothesis vs. situational specificity). That these integrative strategies rest on distinct theoretical foundations requires empirical testing. To what degree do the Trifactor Model and Satellite Model validly characterize the data conditions encountered by scholars in youth development (see also De Los Reyes et al., 2022b)?

Addressing this question requires implementing well-established measurement validation procedures, informed by CONTEXT. Indeed, what if there exist many data conditions in which the Trifactor Model and Satellite Model differ in their performance when used to predict validity criteria (i.e., estimates of score validity)? What if there exists a limited set of data conditions in which the Trifactor Model and Satellite Model perform similarly in terms of score validity? To be clear, addressing these questions does not necessitate a blanket recommendation as to whether researchers ought to implement one model over the other. Rather, addressing these questions requires careful consideration and testing of the "fit" between these strategies and the data conditions to which they may be applied (see also De Los Reyes et al., 2023a). This book provides one set of tests of what we consider a paradigm for evaluating competing models for integrating multi-informant data. The questions these tests address do not speak to specific recommendations on the one integrative model all scholars should use. Rather, this book answers this question: What approach should scholars take when selecting the integrative strategy that best fits the data conditions in which they seek to integrate multi-informant data?

What scholars in youth development require is an approach to guide tests of the validity performance of scores taken from the Trifactor Model and Satellite Model. For these tests to be maximally informative to scholars in youth development, they ought to be grounded in not only theory, but also the data conditions that typify the use of structurally different informants when assessing youth behavior. A key question regarding the use of these integrative strategies remains: How do they perform in tests of the degree to which integrative scores derived from them predict validity criteria? In Chaps. 5, 6, and 7, we address this question with two studies: (a) a Monte Carlo simulation and (b) a real-world test of criterion-related validity.

References

Achenbach, T. M., McConaughy, S. H., & Howell, C. T. (1987). Child/adolescent behavioral and emotional problems: Implications of cross-informant correlations for situational specificity. *Psychological Bulletin, 101*(2), 213–232. https://psycnet.apa.org/doi/10.1037/0033-2909.101.2.213

Al Ghriwati, N., Winter, M. A., Greenlee, J. L., & Thompson, E. L. (2018). Discrepancies between parent and self-reports of adolescent psychosocial symptoms: Associations with family conflict and asthma outcomes. *Journal of Family Psychology, 32*(7), 992–997. https://doi.org/10.1037/fam0000459

Alvarez, I., Herrero, M., Martínez-Pampliega, A., & Escudero, V. (2021). Measuring perceptions of the therapeutic alliance in individual, family, and group therapy from a systemic perspective: Structural validity of the SOFTA-s. *Family Process, 60*(2), 302–315. https://doi.org/10.1111/famp.12565

Armstrong, J. M., Ruttle, P. L., Klein, M. H., Essex, M. J., & Benca, R. M. (2014). Associations of child insomnia, sleep movement, and their persistence with mental health symptoms in childhood and adolescence. *Sleep, 37*(5), 901–909. https://psycnet.apa.org/doi/10.5665/sleep.3656

Bauer, D. J., Howard, A. L., Baldasaro, R. E., Curran, P. J., Hussong, A. M., Chassin, L., & Zucker, R. A. (2013). A trifactor model for integrating ratings across multiple informants. *Psychological Methods, 18*(4), 475–493. https://psycnet.apa.org/doi/10.1037/a0032475

Becker-Haimes, E. M., Jensen-Doss, A., Birmaher, B., Kendall, P. C., & Ginsburg, G. S. (2018). Parent–youth informant disagreement: Implications for youth anxiety treatment. *Clinical Child Psychology and Psychiatry, 23*(1), 42–56. https://doi.org/10.1177/1359104516689586

Boutron, I., Dutton, S., Ravaud, P., & Altman, D. G. (2010). Reporting and interpretation of randomized controlled trials with statistically nonsignificant results for primary outcomes. *JAMA, 303*(20), 2058–2064. https://doi.org/10.1001/jama.2010.651

Campbell, D. T., & Fiske, D. W. (1959). Convergent and discriminant validation by the multitrait-multimethod matrix. *Psychological Bulletin, 56*, 81–105. https://doi.org/10.1037/h0046016

Chen, X., Wang, Y., Li, F., Gong, J., & Yan, Y. (2015). Development and evaluation of the brief sexual openness scale—A construal level theory based approach. *PLoS One, 10*(8), e0136683. https://doi.org/10.1371/journal.pone.0136683

Clark, D. A., Listro, C. J., Lo, S. L., Durbin, C. E., Donnellan, M. B., & Neppl, T. K. (2016). Measurement invariance and child temperament: An evaluation of sex and informant differences on the child behavior questionnaire. *Psychological Assessment, 28*(12), 1646–1662. https://doi.org/10.1037/pas0000299

Clark, D. A., Durbin, C. E., Donnellan, M. B., & Neppl, T. K. (2017). Internalizing symptoms and personality traits color parental reports of child temperament. *Journal of Personality, 85*(6), 852–866. https://doi.org/10.1111/jopy.12293

Curran, P. J., Georgeson, A. R., Bauer, D. J., & Hussong, A. M. (2020). Psychometric models for scoring multiple reporter assessments: Applications to integrative data analysis in prevention science and beyond. *International Journal of Behavioral Development, 45*(1), 40–50. https://doi.org/10.1177/0165025419896620

De Los Reyes, A. (2024). *Discrepant results in mental health research: What they mean, why they matter, and how they inform scientific practices*. Oxford University Press.

De Los Reyes, A., & Epkins, C. C. (2023). Introduction to the special issue. A dozen years of demonstrating that informant discrepancies are more than measurement error: Toward guidelines for integrating data from multi-informant assessments of youth mental health. *Journal of Clinical Child and Adolescent Psychology, 52*(1), 1–18. https://doi.org/10.1080/15374416.2022.2158843

De Los Reyes, A., Henry, D. B., Tolan, P. H., & Wakschlag, L. S. (2009). Linking informant discrepancies to observed variations in young children's disruptive behavior. *Journal of Abnormal Child Psychology, 37*(5), 637–652. https://doi.org/10.1007/s10802-009-9307-3

De Los Reyes, A., Kundey, S. M. A., & Wang, M. (2011). The end of the primary outcome measure: A research agenda for constructing its replacement. *Clinical Psychology Review, 31*(5), 829–838. https://doi.org/10.1016/j.cpr.2011.03.011

De Los Reyes, A., Thomas, S. A., Goodman, K. L., & Kundey, S. M. A. (2013). Principles underlying the use of multiple informants' reports. *Annual Review of Clinical Psychology, 9*, 123–149. https://doi.org/10.1146/annurev-clinpsy-050212-185617

De Los Reyes, A., Augenstein, T. M., Wang, M., Thomas, S. A., Drabick, D. A. G., Burgers, D., & Rabinowitz, J. (2015). The validity of the multi-informant approach to assessing child and adolescent mental health. *Psychological Bulletin, 141*(4), 858–900. https://doi.org/10.1037/a0038498

De Los Reyes, A., Ohannessian, C. M., & Racz, S. J. (2019a). Discrepancies between adolescent and parent reports about family relationships. *Child Development Perspectives, 13*(1), 53–58. https://doi.org/10.1111/cdep.12306

De Los Reyes, A., Lerner, M. D., Keeley, L. M., Weber, R. J., Drabick, D. A., Rabinowitz, J., & Goodman, K. L. (2019b). Improving interpretability of subjective assessments about psychological phenomena: A review and cross-cultural meta-analysis. *Review of General Psychology, 23*(3), 293–319. https://doi.org/10.1177/1089268019837645

De Los Reyes, A., Talbott, E., Power, T., Michel, J., Cook, C. R., Racz, S. J., & Fitzpatrick, O. (2022a). The Needs-to-Goals Gap: How informant discrepancies in youth mental health assessments impact service delivery. *Clinical Psychology Review, 92*, 102114. https://doi.org/10.1016/j.cpr.2021.102114

De Los Reyes, A., Tyrell, F. A., Watts, A. L., & Asmundson, G. J. G. (2022b). Conceptual, methodological, and measurement factors that disqualify use of measurement invariance techniques to detect informant discrepancies in youth mental health assessments. *Frontiers in Psychology, 13*, Article 931296. https://doi.org/10.3389/fpsyg.2022.931296

De Los Reyes, A., Cook, C. R., Sullivan, M., Morrell, N., Hamlin, C., Wang, M., Gresham, F. M., Makol, B. A., Keeley, L. M., & Qasmieh, N. (2022c). The Work and Social Adjustment Scale for Youth: Psychometric properties of the teacher version and evidence of contextual variability in psychosocial impairments. *Psychological Assessment, 34*(8), 777–790. https://doi.org/10.1037/pas0001139

De Los Reyes, A., Wang, M., Lerner, M. D., Makol, B. A., Fitzpatrick, O., & Weisz, J. R. (2023a). The Operations Triad Model and youth mental health assessments: Catalyzing a paradigm shift in measurement validation. *Journal of Clinical Child and Adolescent Psychology, 52*(1), 19–54. https://doi.org/10.1080/15374416.2022.2111684

De Los Reyes, A., Epkins, C. C., Asmundson, G. J. G., Augenstein, T. M., Becker, K. D., Becker, S. P., Bonadio, F. T., Borelli, J. L., Boyd, R. C., Bradshaw, C. P., Burns, G. L., Casale, G., Causadias, J. M., Cha, C. B., Chorpita, B. F., Cohen, J. R., Comer, J. S., Crowell, S. E., Dirks, M. A., et al. (2023b). Editorial statement about *JCCAP*'s 2023 special issue on informant discrepancies in youth mental health assessments: Observations, guidelines, and future directions grounded in 60 years of research. *Journal of Clinical Child and Adolescent Psychology, 52*(1), 147–158. https://doi.org/10.1080/15374416.2022.2158842

Deros, D. E., Racz, S. J., Lipton, M. F., Augenstein, T. M., Karp, J. N., Keeley, L. M., et al. (2018). Multi-informant assessments of adolescent social anxiety: Adding clarity by leveraging reports from unfamiliar peer confederates. *Behavior Therapy, 49*(1), 84–98. https://doi.org/10.1016/j.beth.2017.05.001

Dunning, D., Heath, C., & Suls, J. M. (2004). Flawed self-assessment: Implications for health, education, and the workplace. *Psychological Science in the Public Interest, 5*(3), 69–106. https://doi.org/10.1111/j.1529-1006.2004.00018.x

Edgeworth, F. Y. (1888). The statistics of examinations. *Journal of the Royal Statistical Society, 51*, 598–635. https://www.jstor.org/stable/2339898

Fiske, D. W., & Campbell, D. T. (1992). Citations do not solve problems. *Psychological Bulletin, 112*(3), 393–395. https://doi.org/10.1037/0033-2909.112.3.393

Gardner, T. W., Dishion, T. J., & Connell, A. M. (2008). Adolescent self-regulation as resilience: Resistance to antisocial behavior within the deviant peer context. *Journal of Abnormal Child Psychology, 36*(2), 273–284. https://doi.org/10.1007/s10802-007-9176-6

Grace, R. C. (2001). On the failure of operationism. *Theory and Psychology, 11*(1), 5–33. https://doi.org/10.1177/0959354301111001

Hempel, C. G. (1966). *Philosophy of natural science*. Prentice-Hall.

Highhouse, S. (2009). Designing experiments that generalize. *Organizational Research Methods, 12*(3), 554–566. https://doi.org/10.1177/1094428107300396

Howe, G. W., Dagne, G. A., Brown, C. H., Brincks, A. M., Beardslee, W., Perrino, T., & Pantin, H. (2019). Evaluating construct equivalence of youth depression measures across multiple measures and multiple studies. *Psychological Assessment, 31*(9), 1154–1167. https://doi.org/10.1037/pas0000737

Jungersen, C. M., & Lonigan, C. J. (2021). Do parent and teacher ratings of ADHD reflect the same constructs? A measurement invariance analysis. *Journal of Psychopathology and Behavioral Assessment, 43*(4), 778–792. https://doi.org/10.1007/s10862-021-09874-3

Kraemer, H. C., Measelle, J. R., Ablow, J. C., Essex, M. J., Boyce, W. T., & Kupfer, D. J. (2003). A new approach to integrating data from multiple informants in psychiatric assessment and research: Mixing and matching contexts and perspectives. *American Journal of Psychiatry, 160*(9), 1566–1577. https://doi.org/10.1176/appi.ajp.160.9.1566

Laird, R. D. (2020). Analytical challenges of testing hypotheses of agreement and discrepancy: Comment on Campione-Barr, Lindell, and Giron (2020). *Developmental Psychology, 56*(5), 970–977. https://doi.org/10.1037/dev0000763

Laird, R. D., & De Los Reyes, A. (2013). Testing informant discrepancies as predictors of adolescent psychopathology: Why difference scores cannot tell you what you want to know and how polynomial regression may. *Journal of Abnormal Child Psychology, 41*(1), 1–14. https://doi.org/10.1007/s10802-012-9659-y

Lakind, D., Bradley, W. J., Patel, A., Chorpita, B. F., & Becker, K. D. (2022). A multidimensional examination of the measurement of treatment engagement: Implications for children's mental health services and research. *Journal of Clinical Child and Adolescent Psychology, 51*(4), 453–468. https://doi.org/10.1080/15374416.2021.1941057

Lerner, M. D., De Los Reyes, A., Drabick, D. G., Gerber, A. H., & Gadow, K. D. (2017). Informant discrepancy defines discrete, clinically useful autism spectrum disorder subgroups. *Journal of Child Psychology and Psychiatry, 58*(7), 829–839. https://doi.org/10.1111/jcpp.12730

Makol, B. A. (2022). *Bias versus context models for integrating multi-informant reports of youth mental health* (order no. 28547966). Available from pro Quest Dissertations & Theses Global. (2718669547). https://www.proquest.com/dissertations-theses/bias-versus- context-models-integrating-multi/docview/2718669547/se-2.

Makol, B. A., De Los Reyes, A., Ostrander, R., & Reynolds, E. K. (2019). Parent-youth divergence (and convergence) in reports of youth internalizing problems in psychiatric inpatient care. *Journal of Abnormal Child Psychology, 47*(10), 1677–1689. https://doi.org/10.1007/s10802-019-00540-7

Makol, B. A., Youngstrom, E. A., Racz, S. J., Qasmieh, N., Glenn, L. E., & De Los Reyes, A. (2020). Integrating multiple informants' reports: How conceptual and measurement models may address long-standing problems in clinical decision-making. *Clinical Psychological Science, 8*(6), 953–970. https://doi.org/10.1177/2167702620924439

Murray, A. L., Speyer, L. G., Hall, H. A., Valdebenito, S., & Hughes, C. (2021). Teacher versus parent informant measurement invariance of the strengths and difficulties questionnaire. *Journal of Pediatric Psychology, 46*(10), 1249–1257. https://doi.org/10.1093/jpepsy/jsab062

Olino, T. M., Finsaas, M., Dougherty, L. R., & Klein, D. N. (2018). Is parent–child disagreement on child anxiety explained by differences in measurement properties? An examination of measurement invariance across informants and time. *Frontiers in Psychology, 9*, 1295. https://doi.org/10.3389/fpsyg.2018.01295

Olino, T. M., Michelini, G., Mennies, R. J., Kotov, R., & Klein, D. N. (2021). Does maternal psychopathology bias reports of offspring symptoms? A study using moderated non-linear factor analysis. *Journal of Child Psychology and Psychiatry, 62*(10), 1195–1201. https://doi.org/10.1111/jcpp.13394

Owens, E. B., & Hinshaw, S. P. (2016). Childhood conduct problems and young adult outcomes among women with childhood attention-deficit/hyperactivity disorder (ADHD). *Journal of Abnormal Psychology, 125*(2), 220–232. https://doi.org/10.1037/abn0000084

Richters, J. E. (1992). Depressed mothers as informants about their children: A critical review of the evidence for distortion. *Psychological Bulletin, 112*(3), 485–499. https://doi.org/10.1037/0033-2909.112.3.485

Roberts, B. W., & Caspi, A. (2001). Personality development and the person-situation debate: It's déjà vu all over again. *Psychological Inquiry, 12*(2), 104–109. https://www.jstor.org/stable/1449496

Russell, J. D., Graham, R. A., Neill, E. L., & Weems, C. F. (2016). Agreement in youth-parent perceptions of parenting behaviors: A case for testing measurement invariance in reporter discrepancy research. *Journal of Youth and Adolescence, 45*(10), 2094–2107. https://doi.org/10.1007/s10964-016-0495-1

van der Ende, J., Verhulst, F. C., & Tiemeier, H. (2020). Multitrait-multimethod analyses of change of internalizing and externalizing problems in adolescence: Predicting internalizing and externalizing DSM disorders in adulthood. *Journal of Abnormal Psychology, 129*(4), 343–354. https://doi.org/10.1037/abn0000510

Watts, A. L., Makol, B. A., Palumbo, I. M., De Los Reyes, A., Olino, T. M., Latzman, R. D., DeYoung, C. G., Wood, P. K., & Sher, K. J. (2022). How robust is the p-factor? Using multitrait-multimethod modeling to inform the meaning of general factors of psychopathology in youth. *Clinical Psychological Science, 10*(4), 640–661. https://doi.org/10.1177/21677026211055170

Chapter 5
Monte Carlo Simulation of Strategies for Integrating Behavioral Data in Youth Development

5.1 Study 1 Overview

The value of analytic models and their usage assumptions are dictated by their "fit" to the data conditions to which they will be applied (see also De Los Reyes et al., 2023a; Levy, 1969). It logically follows that implementing analytic models must be guided by a sound theoretical foundation (see Borsboom, 2005). Model implementation must also be guided by a comprehensive set of data—data from not only indices of model fit, but also well-constructed validation studies (e.g., De Los Reyes et al., 2022a; Greene et al., 2022; Revelle, 2024). A hallmark feature of evidence-based assessment calls for data from validation studies to inform researchers' decisions about instrumentation (Hunsley & Mash, 2007; Talbott et al., 2023). Importantly, the use of data to inform decision-making cannot end with the selection of an instrument, particularly if scholars eventually integrate the data produced by that instrument with the data produced by other instruments. What this means is that researchers should also conduct validation tests to probe the data derived from the analytic strategies used to integrate data (De Los Reyes, 2024). These validation studies should test the "fit" between integrative strategies and the data conditions produced by multi-informant assessments (De Los Reyes et al., 2023b).

Consequently, we require research that judges the performance of analytic models when applied to the multi-informant data produced when using structurally different informants. In Chap. 4, we argued that these judgments fall within the purview of validation testing. When it comes to discrepant results, CONTEXT informs these tests. CONTEXT guides users to address questions of direct relevance to making evidence-based decisions about integrative strategies. Under what data conditions do social context models like the Satellite Model optimize the prediction of validity indicators? Conversely, under what data conditions do rater bias models like the Trifactor Model optimize such prediction? As a first step toward addressing these questions, we performed a series of Monte Carlo simulations. We constructed these

B. A. Makol et al., *Youth Development in Context*, Springer Series on Child and Family Studies, https://doi.org/10.1007/978-3-031-80549-3_5

simulations based on prior meta-analytic work on cross-informant correspondence in youth mental health (Achenbach et al., 1987; De Los Reyes et al., 2015). These simulations were also informed by studies indicating that structurally different informants produce discrepant results that often contain domain-relevant data (Fig. 5.1; De Los Reyes & Epkins, 2023; De Los Reyes et al., 2013a, 2022b). Our Monte Carlo simulations estimated the performance of the Trifactor Model and the Satellite Model in terms of their criterion-related validity. Further, these simulations involved modeling a range of data conditions that were based on research in youth mental health and, at the same time, typified behavioral assessments conducted in scholarship in youth development generally. These assessments incorporate reports from structurally different informants. They also produce discrepant results in estimates of behavior—discrepant results that often contain domain-relevant data.

In Fig. 5.2, we graphically depict the parameters used to construct the Monte Carlo simulations. To conservatively test differences in performance between the Satellite Model and the Trifactor Model, we estimated factor parameters for our simulations in ways that mirror the parameters and constraints of the Trifactor Model (see Fig. 2.1). These parameters and constraints informed our construction of data simulations for the external validity criteria. Specifically, the exogenous parameters that we varied across scenarios are the external criteria variance composition (i.e., parameters m, s, and t in Fig. 6.2), the item variance composition (i.e.,

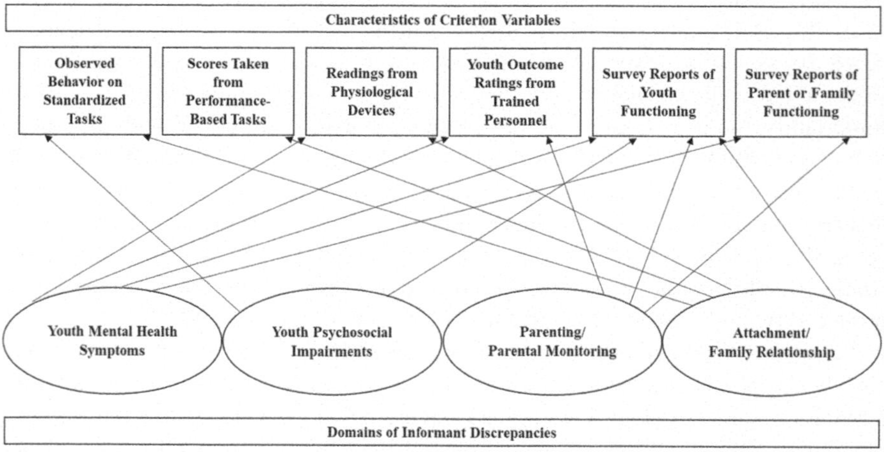

Fig. 5.1 Studies supporting links between discrepant results and domain-relevant criterion variables. *Note*: Citations supporting links described in this figure: Al Ghriwati et al. (2018), Augenstein et al. (2022), Becker-Haimes et al. (2018), Bonadio et al. (2022), Borelli et al. (2016), Charamut et al. (2022), De Los Reyes et al. (2009, 2013b, c, 2016a, b, 2022c), Follet et al. (2023), Human et al. (2016), Humphreys et al. (2017), Laird and De Los Reyes (2013), Lerner et al. (2017), Leung et al. (2016), Luo et al. (2020), Makol and Polo (2018), Makol et al. (2019, 2020, 2021), Nelemans et al. (2016), Nichols and Tanner-Smith (2022), Ohannessian and De Los Reyes (2014), Ohannessian et al. (2016), Okuno et al. (2022), Trang and Yates (2020), Van Heel et al. (2019), Van Petegem et al. (2020), and Zilcha-Mano et al. (2021). (Reproduced from the accepted manuscript version of De Los Reyes & Epkins 2023)

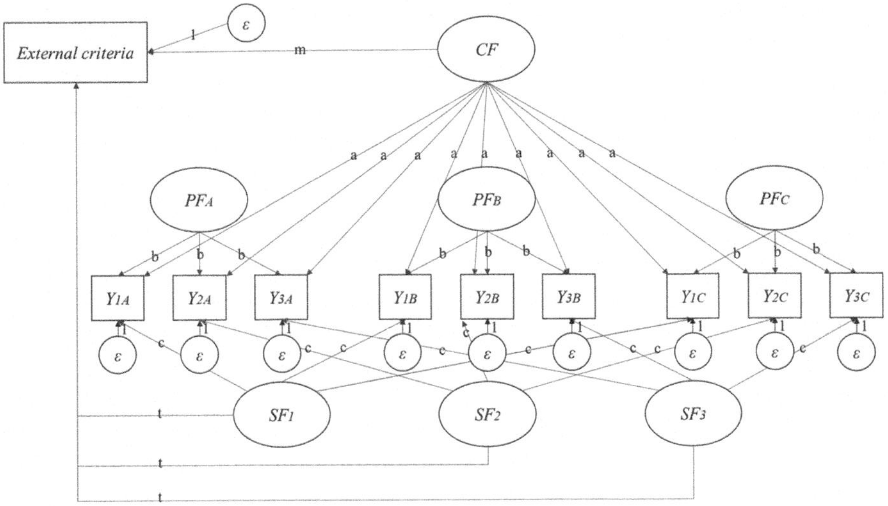

Fig. 5.2 Graphical depiction of parameters used to construct Monte Carlo simulations

parameters a, b, and c in Fig. 5.2), and sample size (i.e., 300 vs. 500, depending on the simulation parameters).

5.2 Study 1 Method

5.2.1 External Criteria Variance Composition

Our composition of external criteria variance consisted of four parameters. First, we modeled random error as the variance of external criteria that information from the three factors cannot explain (i.e., *Common*, *Informant*, and *Item*). We fixed this loading at a value of 1. Second, we modeled the *Common Factor* as a parameter loaded by all items. In Fig. 5.2, we labeled this loading as m, and the variance of external criteria explained by the *Common Factor* is m^2. Third, we modeled *Informant Factors* as analogous to the *Perspective Factors* in the Trifactor Model. These factors capture unique information from informants. In Fig. 5.2, we labeled these loadings as s, and the variance of external criteria explained by *Informant Factors* is three times s^2. Fourth, we modeled *Item Factors* as analogous to the *Specific Factors* in the Trifactor Model. These factors capture unique information from items. In Fig. 5.2, we labeled these loadings as t. The variance of external criteria explained by *Item Factors* is three times t^2. The variances of the external criteria, *Common Factor*, *Informant Factors*, and *Item Factors* were fixed at 1. The variance of external criteria was simulated to be fully explained by random error, *Common Factor*, *Informant Factors*, and *Item Factors*.

5.2.1.1 Simulation of External Criteria Variance Scenarios

We simulated four scenarios in line with the external criteria variance factors (see Table 5.1). First, we simulated a *high random error/Common Factor dominant scenario*, in which we set the variance explained by random error to 0.6, and we set the ratio of variances explained by *Common Factor*, *Informant Factors*, and *Item Factors* to 2:1:1. Second, we simulated a *high random error/all factors equal scenario*, in which we again set the variance explained by random error to 0.6, and we set the ratio of variances explained by *Common Factor*, *Informant Factors*, and *Item Factors* to 1:1:1. Third, we simulated a *low random error/Common Factor dominant scenario*, in which we set the variance explained by random error to 0.3, and we set the ratio of variances explained by *Common Factor*, *Informant Factors*, and *Item Factors* to 2:1:1. Fourth, we simulated a *low random error/all factors equal scenario*, in which we again set the variance explained by random error to 0.3, and we set the ratio of variances explained by *Common Factor*, *Informant Factors*, and *Item Factors* to 1:1:1.

5.2.2 *Item Variance Composition*

Similar to our external criteria variance composition, our composition of item variance consisted of four parameters. First, we modeled random error as the variance of external criteria that the information from the three factors cannot explain. We fixed this loading to 1. Second, we modeled a *Common Factor* with the loading a and with variance in an item explained by the *Common Factor* as a^2. Third, we modeled *Informant Factors* with the loading b and with the variance in an item explained by *Informant Factors* as b^2. Fourth, we modeled *Item Factors* with the loadings c and with the variance in an item explained by *Item Factors* as three times c^2. The variances of the item ratings were fixed at 1 and were fully explained by the random error, *Common Factor*, *Informant Factors*, and *Item Factors*.

5.2.2.1 Simulation of Item Variance Scenarios

We simulated six scenarios in line with the item variance factors described previously (see Table 5.1). First, we simulated a *high random error/Informant Factor dominant scenario*, in which we set the variance explained by random error to 0.6, and we set the ratio of variances explained by the *Common Factor*, *Informant Factors*, and *Item Factors* to 1:2:1. Second, we simulated a *high random error/Common Factor dominant scenario*, in which we again set the variance explained by random error to 0.6, and we set the ratio of variances explained by the *Common Factor*, *Informant Factors*, and *Item Factors* to 2:1:1. Third, we simulated a *high random error/all factors equal scenario*, in which we again set the variance explained by random error to 0.6, and we set the ratio of variances explained by the

Table 5.1 Data structure for Monte Carlo simulation (Study 1)

Scenario	*N*	External criteria variance composition (variance = 1)				Item variance composition (variance = 1)				Commonality	*rs* between informant scale scores	*rs* between informant scale means and external criteria
		Random error	Common factor	Informant factor	Item factor	Random error	Common factor	Informant factor	Item factor			
1	300	0.60	0.20	0.10	0.10	0.60	0.10	0.20	0.10	0.03	0.25	0.38
2	500	0.60	0.20	0.10	0.10	0.60	0.10	0.20	0.10	0.03	0.25	0.38
3	300	0.60	0.20	0.10	0.10	0.60	0.20	0.10	0.10	0.08	0.44	0.43
4	500	0.60	0.20	0.10	0.10	0.60	0.20	0.10	0.10	0.08	0.44	0.43
5	300	0.60	0.20	0.10	0.10	0.60	0.13	0.13	0.13	0.05	0.35	0.41
6	500	0.60	0.20	0.10	0.10	0.60	0.13	0.13	0.13	0.05	0.35	0.41
7	300	0.60	0.20	0.10	0.10	0.30	0.18	0.35	0.18	0.16	0.60	0.50
8	500	0.60	0.20	0.10	0.10	0.30	0.18	0.35	0.18	0.16	0.60	0.50
9	300	0.60	0.20	0.10	0.10	0.30	0.35	0.18	0.18	0.06	0.34	0.45
10	500	0.60	0.20	0.10	0.10	0.30	0.35	0.18	0.18	0.06	0.34	0.45
11	300	0.60	0.20	0.10	0.10	0.30	0.23	0.23	0.23	0.05	0.35	0.41
12	500	0.60	0.20	0.10	0.10	0.30	0.23	0.23	0.23	0.05	0.35	0.41
13	300	0.60	0.13	0.13	0.13	0.60	0.10	0.20	0.10	0.03	0.25	0.38
14	500	0.60	0.13	0.13	0.13	0.60	0.10	0.20	0.10	0.03	0.25	0.38
15	300	0.60	0.13	0.13	0.13	0.60	0.20	0.10	0.10	0.07	0.44	0.41
16	500	0.60	0.13	0.13	0.13	0.60	0.20	0.10	0.10	0.07	0.44	0.41
17	300	0.60	0.13	0.13	0.13	0.60	0.13	0.13	0.13	0.05	0.35	0.40

(continued)

Table 5.1 (continued)

		External criteria variance composition (variance = 1)				Item variance composition (variance = 1)						
Scenario	*N*	Random error	Common factor	Informant factor	Item factor	Random error	Common factor	Informant factor	Item factor	Commonality	*rs* between informant scale scores	*rs* between informant scale means and external criteria
18	500	0.60	0.13	0.13	0.13	0.60	0.13	0.13	0.13	0.05	0.35	0.40
19	300	0.60	0.13	0.13	0.13	0.30	0.18	0.35	0.18	0.14	0.60	0.47
20	500	0.60	0.13	0.13	0.13	0.30	0.18	0.35	0.18	0.14	0.60	0.47
21	300	0.60	0.13	0.13	0.13	0.30	0.35	0.18	0.18	0.06	0.34	0.44
22	500	0.60	0.13	0.13	0.13	0.30	0.35	0.18	0.18	0.06	0.34	0.44
23	300	0.60	0.13	0.13	0.13	0.30	0.23	0.23	0.23	0.05	0.35	0.40
24	500	0.60	0.13	0.13	0.13	0.30	0.23	0.23	0.23	0.05	0.35	0.40
25	300	0.30	0.35	0.18	0.18	0.60	0.10	0.20	0.10	0.05	0.25	0.51
26	500	0.30	0.35	0.18	0.18	0.60	0.10	0.20	0.10	0.05	0.25	0.51
27	300	0.30	0.35	0.18	0.18	0.60	0.20	0.10	0.10	0.14	0.44	0.57
28	500	0.30	0.35	0.18	0.18	0.60	0.20	0.10	0.10	0.14	0.44	0.57
29	300	0.30	0.35	0.18	0.18	0.60	0.13	0.13	0.13	0.10	0.35	0.55
30	500	0.30	0.35	0.18	0.18	0.60	0.13	0.13	0.13	0.10	0.35	0.55
31	300	0.30	0.35	0.18	0.18	0.30	0.18	0.35	0.18	0.27	0.60	0.67
32	500	0.30	0.35	0.18	0.18	0.30	0.18	0.35	0.18	0.27	0.60	0.67
33	300	0.30	0.35	0.18	0.18	0.30	0.35	0.18	0.18	0.11	0.34	0.59
34	500	0.30	0.35	0.18	0.18	0.30	0.35	0.18	0.18	0.11	0.34	0.59
35	300	0.30	0.35	0.18	0.18	0.30	0.23	0.23	0.23	0.10	0.35	0.55
36	500	0.30	0.35	0.18	0.18	0.30	0.23	0.23	0.23	0.10	0.35	0.55

37	300	0.30	0.23	0.23	0.23	0.60	0.10	0.20	0.10	0.10	0.25	0.50
38	500	0.30	0.23	0.23	0.23	0.60	0.10	0.20	0.10	0.10	0.25	0.50
39	300	0.30	0.23	0.23	0.23	0.60	0.20	0.10	0.10	0.12	0.44	0.54
40	500	0.30	0.23	0.23	0.23	0.60	0.20	0.10	0.10	0.12	0.44	0.54
41	300	0.30	0.23	0.23	0.23	0.60	0.13	0.13	0.13	0.09	0.35	0.53
42	500	0.30	0.23	0.23	0.23	0.60	0.13	0.13	0.13	0.09	0.35	0.53
43	300	0.30	0.23	0.23	0.23	0.30	0.18	0.35	0.18	0.24	0.60	0.63
44	500	0.30	0.23	0.23	0.23	0.30	0.18	0.35	0.18	0.24	0.60	0.63
45	300	0.30	0.23	0.23	0.23	0.30	0.35	0.18	0.18	0.11	0.34	0.59
46	500	0.30	0.23	0.23	0.23	0.30	0.35	0.18	0.18	0.11	0.34	0.59
47	300	0.30	0.23	0.23	0.23	0.30	0.23	0.23	0.23	0.09	0.35	0.53
48	500	0.30	0.23	0.23	0.23	0.30	0.23	0.23	0.23	0.09	0.35	0.53

Common Factor, *Informant Factors*, and *Item Factors* to 1:1:1. Fourth, we simulated a *low random error/Informant Factor dominant scenario*, in which we set the variance explained by random error to 0.3, and we set the ratio of variances explained by the *Common Factor*, *Informant Factors*, and *Item Factors* to 1:2:1. Fifth, we simulated a *low random error/Common Factor dominant scenario*, in which we again set the variance explained by random error to 0.3, and we set the ratio of variances explained by the *Common Factor*, *Informant Factors*, and *Item Factors* to 2:1:1. Sixth, we simulated a *low random error/all factors equal scenario*, in which we again set the variance explained by random error to 0.3, and we set the ratio of variances explained by the *Common Factor*, *Informant Factors*, and *Item Factors* to 1:1:1.

5.2.3 Sample Size, Number of Simulation Scenarios, and Number of Simulations per Scenario

Across four external criteria scenarios and six-item variance scenarios, we computed Monte Carlo simulations for two sample size conditions, $N = 300$ and $N = 500$. This totaled 48 scenarios (i.e., 4 * 6 * 2). For each scenario, we computed 1000 Monte Carlo simulations. For each scenario, we estimated the *commonality*—via regression commonality analyses, an estimate of the common or overlapping variance among multiple informants' reports when predicting a common validity criterion (see Cohen et al., 2003; Nimon, 2010). We also estimated the correlations between informant scale means and between informant scale means and external criteria. As noted in Table 5.1, across the 48 scenarios tested, the commonalities varied from 0.03 to 0.24, correlations between informant scale means varied from 0.25 to 0.60, and correlations between informant scale scores and validity criteria varied from 0.38 to 0.67.

The correlations estimated across the 48 scenarios varied as to their representation of "real-world" data conditions in youth mental health research. Yet, collectively, they produced patterns of data that were comparable to key findings from the discrepant results literature. First, the commonalities were aligned with the findings of regression commonality analyses reported by De Los Reyes et al. (2015), which estimated the degree of overlap among parent, teacher, and youth reports on the Achenbach System of Empirically Based Assessments (ASEBAs) in the prediction of a common criterion (i.e., referral status). Second, the correlations between informant scale means were aligned with nationally representative item-level data collected in 2000 and provided to us by the developer of the ASEBA instruments (Thomas M. Achenbach, personal communication, April 29, 2022). Third, the correlations between informant scale means and external criteria were aligned with prior work that estimated relations among informants' reports and independent assessments of observed behavior (Makol et al., 2020).

Taken together, we can consider the 48 scenarios as varying from each other as to their "fit" with the data conditions that typify the use of structurally different informants in youth mental health. Among the 48 scenarios, the estimates from Scenarios 1, 2, 13, and 14 can be seen as the most realistic fit to observations in the discrepant result literature. Specifically, the correlations estimated in these four scenarios were based on the presence of high random error, relatively low *Common Factor* variance, and relatively high *Informant Factor* variance. In fact, within these four scenarios, the estimated commonality (i.e., $r = 0.03$) and mean cross-informant correlation estimate (i.e., $r = 0.25$) track closely with the meta-analytic estimate of cross-informant correspondence reported by Achenbach et al. (1987) and both the cross-informant correspondence and commonality estimates reported in the De Los Reyes et al. (2015) meta-analysis. Similarly, in these scenarios, the estimated mean correlation between informants' reports and external criteria (i.e., $r = 0.38$) is relatively moderate in magnitude. In this sense, this magnitude could be seen as large enough to deem an informant's report as yielding valuable data while at the same time reflective of a magnitude that is near the median of the distribution of correlations observed in Clinical Psychology studies generally (see Schäfer & Schwarz, 2019).

5.2.4 Procedures for Judging the Performance of the Satellite Model and the Trifactor Model

For each of the 48 simulations described previously, we fitted the simulated data to the Trifactor Model and the Satellite Model by computing a series of statistics for both models. We used these statistics and importantly the differences between them to judge the performance of each of these models when predicting external validity criteria. We reported each of these statistics in Table 5.2. Specifically, we computed rates of model convergence for each model, standardized coefficients used to estimate the criterion-related validity performance for each model, and R^2 estimates for total explained variance for each model.

As mentioned previously, the Satellite Model and the Trifactor Model vary in their assumptions regarding unique variance (i.e., discrepant results). However, even if the models vary on the interpretative value they place on information unique to each informant, both models concur on the value of common variance. Thus, for comparative purposes, we based the standardized coefficients and R^2 estimates for each model on the common variance estimate they produce. For the Satellite Model, the standardized coefficient consisted of the standardized regression coefficient of the *Trait* score when regressing external criteria on the *Trait* score, *Context* score, and *Perspective* score. For the Trifactor Model, the standardized coefficient is the standardized regression coefficient of the *Common Factor* on external criteria when regressing external criteria on the *Common Factor*, *Perspective Factor*, and *Specific Factor* in structural equation modeling.

Table 5.2 Results of Monte Carlo simulation (Study 1)

		Satellite model			Trifactor model			Difference		
Scenario	*N*	Convergence rate	*M* of standardized coefficients	*M* of R^2	Convergence rate	*M* of standardized coefficients	*M* of R^2	Convergence rate	*M* of standardized coefficients	*M* of R^2
1	300	100	0.54 (0.04)	0.29 (0.05)	54.0	0.42 (0.10)	0.18 (0.08)	46.0	0.12	0.11
2	500	100	0.54 (0.03)	0.30 (0.03)	80.8	0.44 (0.08)	0.20 (0.07)	19.2	0.10	0.10
3	300	100	0.55 (0.04)	0.30 (0.05)	50.4	0.49 (0.08)	0.25 (0.08)	49.6	0.06	0.05
4	500	100	0.55 (0.03)	0.30 (0.03)	80.8	0.52 (0.07)	0.27 (0.07)	19.2	0.03	0.03
5	300	100	0.55 (0.04)	0.30 (0.05)	59.9	0.46 (0.09)	0.22 (0.08)	40.1	0.09	0.08
6	500	100	0.55 (0.03)	0.30 (0.03)	87.4	0.48 (0.07)	0.23 (0.07)	12.6	0.07	0.07
7	300	100	0.60 (0.04)	0.36 (0.05)	95.9	0.43 (0.10)	0.19 (0.08)	4.1	0.17	0.17
8	500	100	0.60 (0.03)	0.36 (0.03)	99.6	0.44 (0.09)	0.20 (0.07)	0.4	0.16	0.16
9	300	100	0.59 (0.04)	0.35 (0.05)	99.1	0.51 (0.08)	0.27 (0.08)	0.9	0.08	0.08
10	500	100	0.59 (0.03)	0.35 (0.03)	99.9	0.52 (0.07)	0.27 (0.07)	0.1	0.07	0.08
11	300	100	0.60 (0.04)	0.37 (0.05)	98.8	0.47 (0.09)	0.23 (0.08)	1.2	0.13	0.14
12	500	100	0.60 (0.03)	0.37 (0.03)	99.7	0.48 (0.08)	0.23 (0.07)	0.3	0.12	0.14
13	300	100	0.53 (0.04)	0.29 (0.05)	56.1	0.41 (0.11)	0.18 (0.09)	43.9	0.12	0.11

14	500	100	0.53 (0.03)	0.29 (0.03)	83.0	0.43 (0.09)	0.19 (0.08)	17.0	0.10	0.10
15	300	100	0.51 (0.04)	0.26 (0.04)	57.5	0.45 (0.10)	0.21 (0.09)	42.5	0.06	0.05
16	500	100	0.51 (0.03)	0.26 (0.03)	85.3	0.48 (0.09)	0.23 (0.08)	14.7	0.03	0.03
17	300	100	0.53 (0.04)	0.29 (0.04)	64.0	0.44 (0.10)	0.21 (0.09)	36.0	0.09	0.08
18	500	100	0.53 (0.03)	0.29 (0.03)	89.3	0.46 (0.09)	0.22 (0.08)	10.7	0.07	0.07
19	300	100	0.59 (0.04)	0.35 (0.05)	95.8	0.42 (0.10)	0.19 (0.08)	4.2	0.17	0.16
20	500	100	0.59 (0.03)	0.35 (0.03)	99.8	0.43 (0.09)	0.19 (0.08)	0.2	0.16	0.16
21	300	100	0.55 (0.04)	0.31 (0.04)	99.1	0.48 (0.10)	0.24 (0.10)	0.9	0.07	0.07
22	500	100	0.55 (0.03)	0.31 (0.03)	100	0.48 (0.10)	0.24 (0.09)	0	0.07	0.07
23	300	100	0.58 (0.04)	0.34 (0.05)	98.8	0.45 (0.10)	0.21 (0.09)	1.2	0.13	0.13
24	500	100	0.58 (0.03)	0.34 (0.03)	99.4	0.46 (0.09)	0.22 (0.08)	0.6	0.12	0.12
25	300	100	0.72 (0.03)	0.51 (0.04)	59.0	0.57 (0.10)	0.34 (0.12)	41.0	0.15	0.17

(continued)

Table 5.2 (continued)

		Satellite model			Trifactor model			Difference		
Scenario	*N*	Convergence rate	*M* of standardized coefficients	*M* of R^2	Convergence rate	*M* of standardized coefficients	*M* of R^2	Convergence rate	*M* of standardized coefficients	*M* of R^2
26	500	100	0.72 (0.02)	0.51 (0.03)	83.5	0.58 (0.09)	0.35 (0.10)	16.5	0.14	0.16
27	300	100	0.72 (0.03)	0.52 (0.04)	60.0	0.66 (0.09)	0.45 (0.11)	40.0	0.06	0.07
28	500	100	0.72 (0.02)	0.52 (0.03)	86.1	0.69 (0.08)	0.48 (0.10)	13.9	0.03	0.04
29	300	100	0.73 (0.03)	0.53 (0.04)	61.0	0.62 (0.09)	0.39 (0.10)	39.0	0.11	0.14
30	500	100	0.73 (0.02)	0.53 (0.03)	86.9	0.64 (0.07)	0.41 (0.09)	13.1	0.09	0.12
31	300	100	0.79 (0.02)	0.63 (0.04)	95.9	0.58 (0.08)	0.35 (0.09)	4.1	0.21	0.28
32	500	100	0.79 (0.02)	0.63 (0.03)	99.7	0.59 (0.08)	0.35 (0.09)	0.3	0.20	0.28
33	300	100	0.78 (0.02)	0.61 (0.04)	99.3	0.69 (0.08)	0.48 (0.11)	0.7	0.09	0.13
34	500	100	0.78 (0.02)	0.61 (0.03)	99.9	0.69 (0.08)	0.48 (0.11)	0.1	0.09	0.13
35	300	100	0.80 (0.02)	0.64 (0.03)	98.6	0.63 (0.07)	0.41 (0.09)	1.4	0.17	0.13
36	500	100	0.80 (0.02)	0.64 (0.03)	100	0.64 (0.06)	0.41 (0.08)	0	0.16	0.13
37	300	100	0.70 (0.03)	0.50 (0.04)	63.3	0.56 (0.11)	0.33 (0.12)	36.7	0.14	0.17
38	500	100	0.70 (0.02)	0.50 (0.03)	86.0	0.58 (0.10)	0.34 (0.11)	14.0	0.12	0.16

39	300	100	0.68 (0.03)	0.46 (0.04)	66.5	0.61 (0.11)	0.38 (0.13)	33.5	0.07	0.08
40	500	100	0.68 (0.02)	0.46 (0.03)	88.6	0.62 (0.10)	0.39 (0.13)	11.4	0.06	0.07
41	300	100	0.70 (0.03)	0.50 (0.04)	69.1	0.59 (0.11)	0.36 (0.12)	30.9	0.11	0.14
42	500	100	0.71 (0.02)	0.50 (0.03)	91.8	0.61 (0.10)	0.38 (0.12)	8.2	0.10	0.12
43	300	100	0.78 (0.02)	0.61 (0.04)	96.8	0.57 (0.10)	0.34 (0.11)	3.2	0.21	0.27
44	500	100	0.78 (0.02)	0.61 (0.03)	99.9	0.58 (0.10)	0.35 (0.11)	0.1	0.20	0.26
45	300	100	0.73 (0.03)	0.54 (0.04)	99.4	0.62 (0.12)	0.40 (0.15)	0.6	0.11	0.14
46	500	100	0.73 (0.02)	0.54 (0.03)	99.4	0.63 (0.12)	0.41 (0.15)	0.6	0.10	0.13
47	300	100	0.77 (0.02)	0.60 (0.04)	99.1	0.60 (0.10)	0.38 (0.12)	0.9	0.17	0.22
48	500	100	0.77 (0.02)	0.60 (0.03)	99.8	0.61 (0.10)	0.38 (0.12)	0.2	0.16	0.22

For both models, each of the factors is assumed to be orthogonal to one another. As such, standardized coefficients reflect the correlations between the *Trait* score in the Satellite Model (and the *Common Factor* in the Trifactor Model) and external criteria. Similarly, the R^2 estimates reflect the square of the standardized coefficient, and as such, they reflect the proportion of variance in external criteria that can be explained by the *Trait* score in the Satellite Model and the *Common Factor* in the Trifactor Model. Taken together, and to provide as fair a comparison as possible for both models, we judged model performance based on comparisons of standardized coefficients and R^2 estimates.

5.3 Study 1 Results and Discussion

We report the findings from the Monte Carlo simulations in Table 5.2. Each set of findings we report in Table 5.2 refers to the specific parameters modeled in the 48 scenarios described in Table 5.1. To facilitate interpreting findings in Table 5.2, we included the scenario number for each row of findings, which corresponds to the scenarios described in Table 5.1. In this way, readers can interpret the 48 sets of findings reported in Table 5.2 in terms of the models and the parameters simulated for each of the 48 scenarios described in Table 5.1.

The performance of the Satellite Model and the Trifactor Model differed in three respects. First, the convergence rate of the Trifactor Model typically hovered around 50%, a finding that is consistent with prior work. Specifically, studies have varied considerably on whether the Trifactor Model produces adequate model fit, with fit indices often fluctuating, depending on the informants put into the model (cf. Bauer et al., 2013; Clark et al., 2017; Makol, 2022; Martel et al., 2017a, b). In fact, one of the clearest pieces of evidence in support of the Trifactor Model's fit to multi-informant data came from the study by Bauer et al. (2013), in which the model was fit to a pair of informants' reports (i.e., mother and father) who typically display the highest magnitudes of cross-informant correspondence (De Los Reyes et al., 2015). Similarly, for the Trifactor Model, convergence rates from our Monte Carlo simulations tended to be at their highest (i.e., > 95%) when parameter estimates for the *Common Factor* were set at relatively high magnitudes, as well as set higher in magnitude than the *Informant* and *Item Factors*. In contrast, we did not see issues with convergence rates with the Satellite Model. Convergence rates for the Satellite Model were at 100% for all 48 scenarios. Here too, this finding is consistent with prior implementation of the Satellite Model. In fact, adequate model fit indices have been observed (a) using a variety of informants, (b) using varying kinds of instruments, and (c) with sample sizes as low as 60 (e.g., Charamut et al., 2022; De Los Reyes et al., 2022c; Kraemer et al., 2003). In sum, the Satellite Model outperformed the Trifactor Model in terms of providing relatively high convergence rates.

Second, standardized coefficients for the Satellite Model outperformed the Trifactor Model in all 48 scenarios. For the Satellite Model, standardized coefficients for all 48 scenarios were above 0.5 (i.e., the magnitude deemed "large" by

Cohen [1988]), over half were above 0.6, and nearly half were at or above 0.7. In contrast, just over half of the 48 scenarios for the Trifactor Model displayed standardized coefficients above 0.5, less than one-third were above 0.6, and none reached 0.7. Collectively, the differences between the Satellite Model and the Trifactor Model in terms of standardized coefficients ranged from 0.03 to 0.21, with 29 of the 48 scenarios evidencing differences in magnitude at or above 0.10. These 29 scenarios included Scenarios 1, 2, 13, and 14.

Third, similar to the findings for standardized coefficients, the Satellite Model outperformed the Trifactor Model in all 48 scenarios when it came to R^2. For the Satellite Model, 41 of the 48 scenarios were at or above 30% of explained variance, and 22 were at or above 50%. In contrast, only half of the 48 scenarios for the Trifactor Model displayed 30% of explained variance, and none were at or above 50%. Collectively, the differences between the Satellite Model and the Trifactor Model in terms of R^2 ranged from 0.03 to 0.28, with 32 of the 48 scenarios evidencing differences in magnitude at or above 0.10. These 32 scenarios included Scenarios 1, 2, 13, and 14.

5.4 Concluding Comments

Taken together, in Study 1, we found that within data conditions that typify the use of structurally different informants in youth mental health, the Satellite Model and the Trifactor Model exhibited strikingly different levels of performance when predicting validity criteria, with the Satellite Model outperforming the Trifactor Model in every modeling scenario we simulated. Importantly, these simulations cannot be seen as unfairly favoring one integrative strategy over another. Rather, these simulations were based on prior work. We constructed our Monte Carlo simulations using data conditions revealed in authoritative meta-analyses of discrepant results in youth mental health. As such, our simulations displayed parameters that align with (a) typical rates of cross-informant correspondence among informants used in youth mental health assessments (Achenbach et al., 1987), (b) prior work indicating that informants' reports often display little commonality (see De Los Reyes et al., 2015), and (c) prior work indicating that measures of discrepant results predict domain-relevant validity criteria (for a review, see De Los Reyes & Epkins, 2023). Within these data conditions and when estimating correlations between factor scores derived from the models, the Satellite Model consistently and clearly outperformed the Trifactor Model in terms of model convergence, magnitudes of correlations, and amount of explained variance. Nevertheless, an open question is whether we would obtain similar findings when testing the performance of the Trifactor Model and the Satellite Model within real-world data conditions. Chapter 6 describes reasons why "real-world" tests of measurement validation may reveal nuances in the performance of these two integrative strategies, thus setting the stage for Chap. 7, in which we report the findings of just such a validation test.

References

Achenbach, T. M., McConaughy, S. H., & Howell, C. T. (1987). Child/adolescent behavioral and emotional problems: Implications of cross-informant correlations for situational specificity. *Psychological Bulletin, 101*(2), 213–232. https://psycnet.apa.org/doi/10.1037/0033-2909.101.2.213

Al Ghriwati, N., Winter, M. A., Greenlee, J. L., & Thompson, E. L. (2018). Discrepancies between parent and self-reports of adolescent psychosocial symptoms: Associations with family conflict and asthma outcomes. *Journal of Family Psychology, 32*(7), 992–997. https://doi.org/10.1037/fam0000459

Augenstein, T. M., Visser, K. H., Gallagher, K., De Los Reyes, A., D'Angelo, E. A., & Nock, M. K. (2022). Multi-informant reports of depressive symptoms and suicidal ideation among adolescent inpatients. *Suicide and Life-threatening Behavior, 52*(1), 99–109. https://doi.org/10.1111/sltb.12803

Bauer, D. J., Howard, A. L., Baldasaro, R. E., Curran, P. J., Hussong, A. M., Chassin, L., & Zucker, R. A. (2013). A trifactor model for integrating ratings across multiple informants. *Psychological Methods, 18*(4), 475–493. https://psycnet.apa.org/doi/10.1037/a0032475

Becker-Haimes, E. M., Jensen-Doss, A., Birmaher, B., Kendall, P. C., & Ginsburg, G. S. (2018). Parent–youth informant disagreement: Implications for youth anxiety treatment. *Clinical Child Psychology and Psychiatry, 23*(1), 42–56. https://doi.org/10.1177/1359104516689586

Bonadio, F. T., Evans, S. C., Cho, G. Y., Callahan, K. P., Chorpita, B. F., Research Network on Youth Mental Health, & Weisz, J. R. (2022). Whose outcomes come out? Patterns of caregiver- and youth-reported outcomes based on caregiver-youth baseline discrepancies. *Journal of Clinical Child and Adolescent Psychology, 51*(4), 469–483. https://doi.org/10.1080/15374416.2021.1955367

Borelli, J. L., Smiley, P. A., Rasmussen, H. F., & Gómez, A. (2016). Is it about me, you, or us? Stress reactivity correlates of discrepancies in we-talk among parents and preadolescent children. *Journal of Youth and Adolescence, 45*(10), 1996–2010. https://doi.org/10.1007/s10964-016-0459-5

Borsboom, D. (2005). *Measuring the mind.* Cambridge.

Charamut, N. R., Racz, S. J., Wang, M., & De Los Reyes, A. (2022). Integrating multi-informant reports of youth mental health: A construct validation test of Kraemer and colleagues' (2003) Satellite Model. *Frontiers in Psychology, 13*, 911629. https://doi.org/10.3389/fpsyg.2022.911629

Clark, D. A., Durbin, C. E., Donnellan, M. B., & Neppl, T. K. (2017). Internalizing symptoms and personality traits color parental reports of child temperament. *Journal of Personality, 85*(6), 852–866. https://doi.org/10.1111/jopy.12293

Cohen, J. (1988). *Statistical power analysis for the behavioral sciences* (2nd ed.). Erlbaum.

Cohen, J., Cohen, P., West, S. G., & Aiken, L. S. (2003). *Applied multiple regression/correlation analysis for the behavioral sciences* (3rd ed.). Routledge.

De Los Reyes, A. (2024). *Discrepant results in mental health research: What they mean, why they matter, and how they inform scientific practices*. Oxford University Press.

De Los Reyes, A., & Epkins, C. C. (2023). Introduction to the special issue. A dozen years of demonstrating that informant discrepancies are more than measurement error: Toward guidelines for integrating data from multi-informant assessments of youth mental health. *Journal of Clinical Child and Adolescent Psychology, 52*(1), 1–18. https://doi.org/10.1080/15374416.2022.2158843

De Los Reyes, A., Henry, D. B., Tolan, P. H., & Wakschlag, L. S. (2009). Linking informant discrepancies to observed variations in young children's disruptive behavior. *Journal of Abnormal Child Psychology, 37*(5), 637–652. https://doi.org/10.1007/s10802-009-9307-3

De Los Reyes, A., Thomas, S. A., Goodman, K. L., & Kundey, S. M. A. (2013a). Principles underlying the use of multiple informants' reports. *Annual Review of Clinical Psychology, 9*, 123–149. https://doi.org/10.1146/annurev-clinpsy-050212-185617

De Los Reyes, A., Lerner, M. D., Thomas, S. A., Daruwala, S. E., & Goepel, K. A. (2013b). Discrepancies between parent and adolescent beliefs about daily life topics and performance on an emotion recognition task. *Journal of Abnormal Child Psychology, 41*(6), 971–982. https://doi.org/10.1007/s10802-013-9733-0

De Los Reyes, A., Salas, S., Menzer, M. M., & Daruwala, S. E. (2013c). Criterion validity of interpreting scores from multi-informant statistical interactions as measures of informant discrepancies in psychological assessments of children and adolescents. *Psychological Assessment, 25*(2), 509–519. https://doi.org/10.1037/a0032081

De Los Reyes, A., Augenstein, T. M., Wang, M., Thomas, S. A., Drabick, D. A. G., Burgers, D., & Rabinowitz, J. (2015). The validity of the multi-informant approach to assessing child and adolescent mental health. *Psychological Bulletin, 141*(4), 858–900. https://doi.org/10.1037/a0038498

De Los Reyes, A., Alfano, C. A., Lau, S., Augenstein, T. M., & Borelli, J. L. (2016a). Can we use convergence between caregiver reports of adolescent mental health to index severity of adolescent mental health concerns? *Journal of Child and Family Studies, 25*(1), 109–123. https://doi.org/10.1007/s10826-015-0216-5

De Los Reyes, A., Ohannessian, C. M., & Laird, R. D. (2016b). Developmental changes in discrepancies between adolescents' and their mothers' views of family communication. *Journal of Child and Family Studies, 25*(3), 790–797. https://doi.org/10.1007/s10826-015-0275-7

De Los Reyes, A., Talbott, E., Power, T., Michel, J., Cook, C. R., Racz, S. J., & Fitzpatrick, O. (2022a). The Needs-to-Goals Gap: How informant discrepancies in youth mental health assessments impact service delivery. *Clinical Psychology Review, 92*, Article 102114. https://doi.org/10.1016/j.cpr.2021.102114

De Los Reyes, A., Tyrell, F. A., Watts, A. L., & Asmundson, G. J. G. (2022b). Conceptual, methodological, and measurement factors that disqualify use of measurement invariance techniques to detect informant discrepancies in youth mental health assessments. *Frontiers in Psychology, 13*, Article 931296. https://doi.org/10.3389/fpsyg.2022.931296

De Los Reyes, A., Cook, C. R., Sullivan, M., Morrell, N., Hamlin, C., Wang, M., Gresham, F. M., Makol, B. A., Keeley, L. M., & Qasmieh, N. (2022c). The Work and Social Adjustment Scale for Youth: Psychometric properties of the teacher version and evidence of contextual variability in psychosocial impairments. *Psychological Assessment, 34*(8), 777–790. https://doi.org/10.1037/pas0001139

De Los Reyes, A., Wang, M., Lerner, M. D., Makol, B. A., Fitzpatrick, O., & Weisz, J. R. (2023a). The Operations Triad Model and youth mental health assessments: Catalyzing a paradigm shift in measurement validation. *Journal of Clinical Child and Adolescent Psychology, 52*(1), 19–54. https://doi.org/10.1080/15374416.2022.2111684

De Los Reyes, A., Epkins, C. C., Asmundson, G. J. G., Augenstein, T. M., Becker, K. D., Becker, S. P., Bonadio, F. T., Borelli, J. L., Boyd, R. C., Bradshaw, C. P., Burns, G. L., Casale, G., Causadias, J. M., Cha, C. B., Chorpita, B. F., Cohen, J. R., Comer, J. S., Crowell, S. E., Dirks, M. A., et al. (2023b). Editorial statement about *JCCAP*'s 2023 special issue on informant discrepancies in youth mental health assessments: Observations, guidelines, and future directions grounded in 60 years of research. *Journal of Clinical Child and Adolescent Psychology, 52*(1), 147–158. https://doi.org/10.1080/15374416.2022.2158842

Follet, L., Okuno, H., & De Los Reyes, A. (2023). Assessing peer-related impairments linked to adolescent social anxiety: Strategic selection of informants optimizes prediction of clinically relevant domains. *Behavior Therapy, 54*(1), 29–42. https://doi.org/10.1016/j.beth.2022.06.010

Greene, A. L., Eaton, N. R., Forbes, M. K., Fried, E. I., Watts, A. L., Kotov, R., & Krueger, R. F. (2022). Model fit is a fallible indicator of model quality in quantitative psychopathology research: A reply to Bader and Moshagen. *Journal of Psychopathology and Clinical Science, 131*(6), 696–703. https://doi.org/10.1037/abn0000770

Human, L. J., Dirks, M. A., DeLongis, A., & Chen, E. (2016). Congruence and incongruence in adolescents' and parents' perceptions of the family: Using response surface analysis to examine links with adolescents' psychological adjustment. *Journal of Youth and Adolescence, 45*(10), 2022–2035. https://doi.org/10.1007/s10964-016-0517-z

Humphreys, K. L., Weems, C. F., & Scheeringa, M. S. (2017). The role of anxiety control and treatment implications of informant agreement on child PTSD symptoms. *Journal of Clinical Child and Adolescent Psychology, 46*(6), 903–914. https://doi.org/10.1080/15374416.2015.1094739

Hunsley, J., & Mash, E. J. (2007). Evidence-based assessment. *Annual Review of Clinical Psychology, 3*, 29–51. https://doi.org/10.1146/annurev.clinpsy.3.022806.091419

Kraemer, H. C., Measelle, J. R., Ablow, J. C., Essex, M. J., Boyce, W. T., & Kupfer, D. J. (2003). A new approach to integrating data from multiple informants in psychiatric assessment and research: Mixing and matching contexts and perspectives. *American Journal of Psychiatry, 160*(9), 1566–1577. https://doi.org/10.1176/appi.ajp.160.9.1566

Laird, R. D., & De Los Reyes, A. (2013). Testing informant discrepancies as predictors of adolescent psychopathology: Why difference scores cannot tell you what you want to know and how polynomial regression may. *Journal of Abnormal Child Psychology, 41*(1), 1–14. https://doi.org/10.1007/s10802-012-9659-y

Lerner, M. D., De Los Reyes, A., Drabick, D. G., Gerber, A. H., & Gadow, K. D. (2017). Informant discrepancy defines discrete, clinically useful autism spectrum disorder subgroups. *Journal of Child Psychology and Psychiatry, 58*(7), 829–839. https://doi.org/10.1111/jcpp.12730

Leung, J. T., Shek, D. T., & Li, L. (2016). Mother–child discrepancy in perceived family functioning and adolescent developmental outcomes in families experiencing economic disadvantage in Hong Kong. *Journal of Youth and Adolescence, 45*(10), 2036–2048. https://doi.org/10.1007/s10964-016-0469-3

Levy, P. (1969). Platonic true scores and rating scales: A case of uncorrelated definitions. *Psychological Bulletin, 71*(4), 276–277. https://doi.org/10.1037/h0026855

Luo, R., Chen, F., Yuan, C., Ma, X., & Zhang, C. (2020). Parent–child discrepancies in perceived parental favoritism: Associations with children's internalizing and externalizing problems in Chinese families. *Journal of Youth and Adolescence, 49*(1), 60–73. https://doi.org/10.1007/s10964-019-01148-2

Makol, B. A. (2022). *Bias versus context models for integrating multi-informant reports of youth mental health* (order no. 28547966). Available from ProQuest Dissertations & Theses Global. (2718669547). https://www.proquest.com/dissertations-theses/bias-versus- context-models-integrating-multi/docview/2718669547/se-2

Makol, B. A., & Polo, A. J. (2018). Parent-child endorsement discrepancies among youth at chronic-risk for depression. *Journal of Abnormal Child Psychology, 46*(5), 1077–1088. https://doi.org/10.1007/s10802-017-0360-z

Makol, B. A., De Los Reyes, A., Ostrander, R., & Reynolds, E. K. (2019). Parent-youth divergence (and convergence) in reports of youth internalizing problems in psychiatric inpatient care. *Journal of Abnormal Child Psychology, 47*(10), 1677–1689. https://doi.org/10.1007/s10802-019-00540-7

Makol, B. A., Youngstrom, E. A., Racz, S. J., Qasmieh, N., Glenn, L. E., & De Los Reyes, A. (2020). Integrating multiple informants' reports: How conceptual and measurement models may address long-standing problems in clinical decision-making. *Clinical Psychological Science, 8*(6), 953–970. https://doi.org/10.1177/2167702620924439

Makol, B. A., De Los Reyes, A., Garrido, E., Harlaar, N., & Taussig, H. (2021). Assessing the mental health of maltreated youth with child welfare involvement using multi-informant reports. *Child Psychiatry and Human Development, 52*(1), 49–62. https://doi.org/10.1007/s10578-020-00985-8

Martel, M. M., Markon, K., & Smith, G. T. (2017a). Research review: Multi-informant integration in child and adolescent psychopathology diagnosis. *Journal of Child Psychology and Psychiatry, 58*(2), 116–128. https://doi.org/10.1111/jcpp.12611

Martel, M. M., Nigg, J. T., & Schimmack, U. (2017b). Psychometrically informed approach to integration of multiple informant ratings in adult ADHD in a community-recruited sample. *Assessment, 24*(3), 279–289. https://doi.org/10.1177/1073191116646443

Nelemans, S. A., Branje, S. J., Hale, W. W., Goossens, L., Koot, H. M., Oldehinkel, A. J., & Meeus, W. H. (2016). Discrepancies between perceptions of the parent–adolescent relationship and early adolescent depressive symptoms: An illustration of polynomial regression analysis. *Journal of Youth and Adolescence, 45*(10), 2049–2063. https://doi.org/10.1007/s10964-016-0503-5

Nichols, L. M., & Tanner-Smith, E. E. (2022). Discrepant parent-adolescent reports of parenting practices: Associations with adolescent internalizing and externalizing symptoms. *Journal of Youth and Adolescence, 51*(6), 1153–1168. https://doi.org/10.1007/s10964-022-01601-9

Nimon, K. (2010). Regression commonality analysis: Demonstration of an SPSS solution. *Multiple Linear Regression Viewpoints, 36*, 10–17. http://mlrv.ua.edu/2010/vol36_1/nimon_proof_2.pdf

Ohannessian, C. M., & De Los Reyes, A. (2014). Discrepancies in adolescents' and their mothers' perceptions of the family and adolescent anxiety symptomatology. *Parenting: Science and Practice, 14*(1), 1–18. https://doi.org/10.1080/15295192.2014.870009

Ohannessian, C. M., Laird, R. D., & De Los Reyes, A. (2016). Discrepancies in adolescents' and their mother's perceptions of the family and mothers' psychological symptomatology. *Journal of Youth and Adolescence, 45*(10), 2011–2021. https://doi.org/10.1007/s10964-016-0477-3

Okuno, H., Rezeppa, T., Raskin, T., & De Los Reyes, A. (2022). Adolescent safety behaviors and social anxiety: Links to psychosocial impairments and functioning with unfamiliar peer confederates. *Behavior Modification, 46*(6), 1314–1345. https://doi.org/10.1177/01454455211054019

Revelle, W. (2024). The seductive beauty of latent variable models: Or why I don't believe in the Easter bunny. *Personality and Individual Differences, 221*, 112552. https://doi.org/10.1016/j.paid.2024.112552

Schäfer, T., & Schwarz, M. A. (2019). The meaningfulness of effect sizes in psychological research: Differences between sub-disciplines and the impact of potential biases. *Frontiers in Psychology, 10*, 813. https://doi.org/10.3389/fpsyg.2019.00813

Talbott, E., De Los Reyes, A., Kearns, D. M., Mancilla-Martinez, J., Cook, C. R., & Wang, M. (2023). Evidence-based assessment in special education research: Advancing the use of evidence in assessment tools and empirical processes. *Exceptional Children, 89*(4), 467–487. https://doi.org/10.1177/00144029231171092

Trang, D. T., & Yates, T. M. (2020). (in)congruent parent–child reports of parental behaviors and later child outcomes. *Journal of Child and Family Studies, 29*(7), 1845–1860. https://doi.org/10.1007/s10826-020-01733-1

Van Heel, M., Bijttebier, P., Colpin, H., Goossens, L., Van Den Noortgate, W., Verschueren, K., & Van Leeuwen, K. (2019). Adolescent-parent discrepancies in perceptions of parenting: Associations with adolescent externalizing problem behavior. *Journal of Child and Family Studies, 28*(11), 3170–3182. https://doi.org/10.1007/s10826-019-01493-7

Van Petegem, S., Antonietti, J. P., Eira Nunes, C., Kins, E., & Soenens, B. (2020). The relationship between maternal overprotection, adolescent internalizing and externalizing problems, and psychological need frustration: A multi-informant study using response surface analysis. *Journal of Youth and Adolescence, 49*(1), 162–177. https://doi.org/10.1007/s10964-019-01126-8

Zilcha-Mano, S., Shimshoni, Y., Silverman, W. K., & Lebowitz, E. R. (2021). Parent-child agreement on family accommodation differentially predicts outcomes of child-based and parent-based child anxiety treatment. *Journal of Clinical Child and Adolescent Psychology, 50*(3), 427–439. https://doi.org/10.1080/15374416.2020.1756300

Chapter 6
Situational Specificity, Validity Criteria, and the Design of Measurement Validation Studies in Youth Development

This chapter returns to the notion of situational specificity advanced by Achenbach et al. (1987), which we first learned about in Chap. 1. Recall a core element of this notion—discrepant results may index how youth behavior changes across social contexts relevant to their day-to-day lives. The fact that youth demonstrate differences in how they behave across contexts has a cascading effect on all aspects of how we understand youth behavior, including how to implement interventions to change youth behavior, such as mental health concerns (see De Los Reyes et al., 2017a, 2022a, b). The reality that youth often behave differently depending on where they are necessitates the use of structurally different informants, particularly those whose observations of youth are often localized to specific contexts (e.g., parent at home vs. teacher at school). Yet this level of context sensitivity is insufficient to truly make sense of the behavioral data that scholars in youth development collect.

Prior work highlights that even when implementing sophisticated analytic strategies such as structural equation modeling, the discrepancies observed among multi-informant data are uninterpretable if all data came from instruments based on the same measurement modality, such as the use of parallel surveys across informants (see Watts et al., 2022). Stated another way, in the presence of *shared method biases* or *criterion contamination* (see also Garb, 2003; Hunsley & Meyer, 2003; Smith et al., 2003), one cannot distinguish discrepant results that are domain-relevant from those that reflect measurement confounds. Valid approaches to assessing youth behavior require more than structurally different informants—they require independent validity indicators to make sense of the data produced by these informants' reports.

To understand the importance of independent validity indicators, let us consider the use of these indicators when scholars seek to design interventions to change youth behavior. For instance, the intervention models that factor into the delivery of youth mental health services—such as classical conditioning, cognitive theory, radical behaviorism, and social learning theory (Bandura, 1977; Beck, 1993; Rescorla

B. A. Makol et al., *Youth Development in Context*, Springer Series on Child and Family Studies, https://doi.org/10.1007/978-3-031-80549-3_6

& Wagner, 1972; Skinner, 1953)—each hinge on adapting therapeutic techniques (e.g., cognitive restructuring, therapeutic exposures, token economies, homework activities) to the unique contexts that are germane to the mental health concerns of youth who receive services (e.g., home, school, peer interactions; Alfano & Beidel, 2011; Sewart & Craske, 2020; Weisz & Kazdin, 2017). Let us consider the use of assessment data to inform decision-making surrounding who ought to receive these services, which specific services should be implemented, and determining whether the services are producing positive benefits among the youth who receive them. If youth behavior must be understood as it manifests within specific contexts, and the services youth receive are tailored to their unique needs, then assessments designed to understand the nature and course of these services must also be context-sensitive (see also De Los Reyes et al., 2022a).

The connections among the notion of situational specificity, the context-sensitivity of youth behavior, and the assessments used to understand this behavior have support from controlled experimentation (see De Los Reyes et al., 2023a). This experiment involved developing videotaped simulations of items contained in a widely used measure of social skills, the Social Skills Improvement System—Rating Scales (SSIS-RS; Gresham et al., 2010). A pretest sample of these items ensured that they accurately simulated the items they were designed to represent. Following this pretest, an independent sample of participants was randomly assigned to two groups. Each group observed a set of videotaped behaviors that the other did not. Each group also observed a common set of behaviors. In this way, the experiment exposed each group to behaviors that were context-specific as well as behaviors that were cross-contextual. Following this observational period, the participants completed a "behavioral checklist" that prompted them to endorse whether they viewed the behaviors described in the items. The behaviors described in the checklist included all the behaviors observed by the two groups, along with a set of behaviors that neither group observed (i.e., to allow for making "false positive" ratings for behaviors that clearly were not observed). As seen in Table 6.1, the study revealed large effects for context sensitivity, namely, distinct patterns of reports for each group who viewed behaviors that the other group did not. The study also revealed near-zero differences between groups on both behaviors that every participant observed as well as behaviors that none observed. This experiment supports the idea that situational specificity in youth behavior can cause informants to produce large, variant response patterns in behavioral ratings.

Situational specificity and its implications for interpreting behavioral data collected by scholars in youth development prompt us to consider the Monte Carlo simulations reported in Chap. 5. These simulations did not account for a core feature of research practices in youth development. In youth development, scholars require multi-modal indicators to distinguish discrepant results that contain valid data from those that reflect measurement confounds (see De Los Reyes, 2024; Makol et al., 2020; Talbott et al., 2023; Watts et al., 2022). Along these lines, CONTEXT allows its users to detect valid data using the structural differences among informants, not just data from informants' responses on instruments. Yet, how do users of CONTEXT detect these valid discrepant results? This chapter

Table 6.1 Between-group differences in identification probabilities of videotaped social skill behavior, as a function of variations in situational specificity

Behaviors observed by experimental groups	Group N	Mean probabilities of video identification	Standard deviations (SD) of video identification	Effect sizes of mean differences reflecting situational specificity
Videotaped behaviors observed by Group 1 and not Group 2 (n = 10 items)	Group 1 N: 87 Group 2 N: 95	Group 1 mean: 74.71 Group 2 mean: 22.00	Group 1 SD: 20.79 Group 2 SD: 21.42	Cohen's d: +2.50
Videotaped behaviors observed by Group 2 and not Group 1 (n = 10 items)	Group 1 N: 87 Group 2 N: 95	Group 1 mean: 29.08 Group 2 mean: 79.16	Group 1 SD: 18.40 Group 2 SD: 17.11	Cohen's d: −2.82
Videotaped behaviors observed by both groups (n = 15 items)	Group 1 N: 87 Group 2 N: 95	Group 1 mean: 89.43 Group 2 mean: 90.11	Group 1 SD: 13.08 Group 2 SD: 13.11	Cohen's d: −0.05
Behaviors observed by neither group (n = 85 items)	Group 1 N: 87 Group 2 N: 95	Group 1 mean: 20.07 Group 2 mean: 18.25	Group 1 SD: 12.85 Group 2 SD: 14.24	Cohen's d: +0.13

Note: reproduced from the accepted manuscript version of De Los Reyes et al. (2023a)

addresses this larger question by linking situational specificity to the research practices that guide selections of validity criteria and study design in youth development. In the process, we describe the design of Study 2, a measurement validation study designed to probe the performance of the Trifactor Model and the Satellite Model in terms of criterion-related validity. This chapter describes Study 2's design, with the goal of setting the stage for reporting the study's results in Chap. 7.

6.1 Context-Sensitive Validity Criteria

Understanding discrepant results requires the use of assessments that are sensitive to the social contexts in which youth behave. This includes the use of multiple informants whose reports are based on observations of youth behavior within and across various domain-relevant social contexts, such as home and school. To make sense of the data produced by these reports, this also includes the use of independent validity criteria. Consistent with situational specificity, a core feature of these validity criteria is that they, like informants' reports, are context-sensitive in how they index youth behavior. What characteristics must scholars keep in mind when selecting these validity criteria? To address this question, let us consider how CONTEXT guides users in the criteria selection process.

The criterion-related validity approach taken within CONTEXT involves the use of validity criteria that harbor two characteristics. First, the validity criteria contain structural characteristics of their own, namely, they reference the functioning of those undergoing evaluation, and within contexts that are relevant to understanding their behavior. Along these lines, a long-held tradition of scholarship in youth development involves the use of structurally different tasks and procedures designed to understand youth behavior as it manifests in social contexts relevant to everyday life. Consider Table 6.2, which provides examples of these kinds of tasks. They include naturalistic home and school observations, scores on academic achievement tests, and controlled laboratory observations of social interactions. In essence, just as the Satellite Model calls for "mixing and matching" informants relative to their own contexts of observation, CONTEXT calls for strategically selecting validity criteria to detect links between patterns of multi-informant data and specific contexts that are germane to understanding the behavior of the youth undergoing evaluation. Recall the discussion that opened this chapter, which highlighted the context-sensitive nature of intervention models. In line with these intervention models, the use of context-sensitive validity criteria not only aligns with CONTEXT-informed measurement validation procedures, but also with how instrumentation is used in research and service settings to understand behavior (e.g., see also Cannon et al., 2020; De Los Reyes & Aldao, 2015; De Los Reyes et al., 2019a, b, c; Groth-Marnat & Wright, 2016; Wakschlag et al., 2010).

Table 6.2 Examples of context-sensitive validity criteria using methods other than informants' surveys

Authors and publication year	Context	Brief description	Examples of methods used
Donenberg and Weisz (1997); Gunnar et al. (2009); Kiecolt-Glaser et al. (2005); Thomas et al. (2019)	Discussions between significant others (e.g., between parents and youth, between caregivers)	Dyadic interactions between significant others, in which the experimenter selects topics for dyads to discuss, with the general task of "coming to a resolution" on the topic discussed (chores, in-laws, spending time with family)	Independent observers, peripheral physiology, saliva tests, wound healing
Beidel et al. (2010); Cannon et al. (2020); DeWall et al. (2010); Silk et al. (2012)	Laboratory-controlled interactions between unfamiliar people	Virtual (e.g., video games, Internet chatroom) or in vivo interactions between participants and unfamiliar people (i.e., typically same-age peers) that expose participants to social situations that may provoke aversive reactions	Independent observers, peripheral physiology, saliva tests, ecological momentary assessment data, neuroimaging
Benner et al. (2022); De Los Reyes et al. (2022c); Fanger et al. (2012); Vlachou et al. (2014)	Naturalistic classroom observations	Trained observers enter classrooms or other academic settings (e.g., recess) and directly observe how participants behave within these settings, in as much of an unobtrusive manner as possible	Independent observers

(continued)

Table 6.2 (continued)

Authors and publication year	Context	Brief description	Examples of methods used
d'Apice et al. (2019); Bousha and Twentyman (1984); Steinglass (1979); Tesh and Holditch-Davis (1997)	Naturalistic home observations	Trained observers enter the home and directly observe how participants behave within this setting, in as much of an unobtrusive manner as possible	Independent observers
De Los Reyes, Aldao, et al. (2017b); Glenn et al. (2019); Mian et al. (2015); Wakschlag et al. (2008)	Cross-contextual behavioral tasks	Controlled laboratory observations of how participants behave when completing tasks and/or interacting with various people; activities are selected under the pretense that they may produce contextual variations in behavior	Independent observers, peripheral physiology
Beidel et al. (1989); Bouma et al. (2009); Dickerson and Kemeny (2004); Gunnar et al. (2009)	Impromptu speech tasks	Participants are instructed to give a speech about a predefined topic or set of topics and/or a topic of their choosing, typically to an audience of personnel trained to react to the speech in stress-provoking ways (e.g., neutral facial expressions, verbal prompts to speed up their speech)	Independent observers, peripheral physiology, saliva tests
Lakind et al. (2022); Makol et al. (2019); Marci et al. (2007); McLeod et al. (2023)	Characteristics of treatment delivered in a controlled setting	Independent assessments of features of treatment response or treatment processes, such as treatment integrity, treatment engagement, therapeutic relationship, therapist empathy, and treatment modalities	Independent observers, peripheral physiology
Jeon and Yamashito (2014); Lin et al. (2021); Pascual et al. (2019); Zhang and Zhang (2022)	Standardized tests delivered in an academic setting	Tests administered in academic settings that evaluate performance on such academic domains as reading comprehension, vocabulary knowledge, math performance, and academic achievement	Independent evaluators
Daley et al. (2003); Hooley and Parker (2006); McCarty and Weisz (2002); Sher-Censor (2015)	Expressed emotion between significant others	5-min speech sample, in which participant is prompted to speak about a relative who experiences mental health concerns	Independent evaluators

Let us consider a second characteristic of the validity criteria used in CONTEXT-informed approaches to testing criterion-related validity. As mentioned previously, prior work highlights that even when using context-sensitive validity criteria and structurally different informants, the use of multi-modal approaches to assess youth behavior makes all the difference in drawing valid inferences from assessment results and study findings (see Makol et al., 2020; Watts et al., 2022). Thus, a hallmark feature of CONTEXT-aligned validation studies involves the use of validity criteria that are not only context-sensitive but also independent in measurement modality, relative to the modalities typically used to collect multi-informant data (see De Los Reyes et al., 2023a, b). Examples of these measurement modalities include performance-based tests, passive data from mobile computing devices (e.g., location data), physiological readings from wearable devices (e.g., heart rate data from a wristwatch monitor), and ratings from trained research personnel.

Collectively, the two validity criteria characteristics we described necessitate measurement validation studies, to complement the findings from the Monte Carlo simulations conducted as part of Study 1. Indeed, CONTEXT-aligned validity studies are well positioned to address the realities of measurement validation when using structurally different informants. Specifically, validating data from structurally different informants necessitates context-sensitive validity criteria. If so, then validity criteria, though independent in method, will nonetheless overlap in contexts of observation more so with some informants rather than others. For example, a naturalistic observation of how a child behaves at school, by construction, will produce data that align more so with teachers' reports than they do with parents' reports. Alternatively, a controlled observation of how an adolescent interacts with peers will produce data that align more so with peers' reports than they do with parents' reports and vice versa for naturalistic observations of how that adolescent interacts with caregivers at home. This is not a limitation of any one assessment approach per se. For instance, in scholarship in youth mental health, evidence-based approaches to delivering context-sensitive mental health services necessitate the use of evidence that is also context-sensitive (De Los Reyes et al., 2022a). Yet it does create the potential for informants to vary in their ability to predict validity criteria. How do the Satellite Model and the Trifactor Model perform under these conditions, in which informants' reports may vary in their ability to predict context-sensitive validity criteria? Study 2 addressed this question in a way that complements what we learned from Study 1's findings.

6.2 Study 2 Method

6.2.1 Participants and Procedures

We addressed our Study 2 aims using the data from a well-characterized study—*Project CONTEXT* (see De Los Reyes, 2024). The design of Project CONTEXT facilitates addressing questions regarding the psychometric properties of scores taken from instruments used to assess adolescent mental health. As such, scores taken from the instruments used in Project CONTEXT have been thoroughly tested in terms of their psychometric properties. These tests consist of measurement validation studies that have leveraged a host of not only measurement modalities but also data sources, which include caregivers, adolescents, and both trained and untrained observers. In Table 6.3, we report studies and main findings from all published work on Project CONTEXT to date, which totals over 20 peer-reviewed journal articles.

We recruited adolescents and caregivers within the regions of Maryland, Washington, DC, and northern Virginia. Participant recruitment began in April 2014 and ended in late February 2020, in line with COVID-19 restriction guidelines for on-campus participant recruitment at the University of Maryland—the site where the study took place. Recruitment methods included online advertisements (e.g., Craigslist) and flyers posted in local businesses (e.g., libraries, pediatricians' office). Participants responded to one of two posted advertisements: (a) a study providing a no-cost clinical social anxiety evaluation for adolescents (i.e., *clinic-referred adolescents*) and (b) a nonclinical study on family relationships (i.e., *community-control adolescents*). The method we used to advertise the study and recruit participants was the only way in which participants varied as to study procedures. That is, we held all study procedures consistent across participants, regardless of recruitment strategy. This included the survey battery that participants completed, as well as the interactions between adolescents and personnel trained to behave as same-age, unfamiliar peers (i.e., peer confederates). These peer confederates interacted with

Table 6.3 Peer-reviewed publications to date using data from project CONTEXT, organized chronologically ($N = 24$)

Authors and publication year	Survey data sources	Instrumentation	Validity criteria	Summary of main findings
Rausch et al. (2017)	A, Ca	Surveys, controlled observations	Surveys of adolescent functioning, self-reported arousal within interactions with unfamiliar peers	Adolescents and caregivers provide psychometrically sound reports on the Beck Depression Inventory-II (BDI-II); only adolescents' self-reports on the BDI-II predicted adolescents' arousal within interactions with unfamiliar peers
Beale et al. (2018)	A, Ca	Surveys	Surveys of adolescent functioning	Using a short list of three items assessing peer-related impairments (number of friends, trouble making friends, and trouble keeping friends), one can efficiently screen for peer-related impairments of specific relevance to adolescent social anxiety

(continued)

Table 6.3 (continued)

Authors and publication year	Survey data sources	Instrumentation	Validity criteria	Summary of main findings
Deros et al. (2018)	A, Ca, PC	Surveys, controlled observations	Surveys of adolescent functioning, self-reported arousal within interactions with unfamiliar peers	Adolescents' social anxiety reports correlated with reports on parallel measures from caregivers in the .30 s and with peer confederates in the .40 s to .50 s, whereas reports from caregiver-confederate dyads correlated in the 0.07 to 0.22 range Adolescent, caregiver, and peer confederate social anxiety reports related to reports on trait measures of adolescent social anxiety and depressive symptoms and distinguished adolescents on referral status. Confederates' social anxiety reports incrementally predicted adolescents' self-reported social anxiety over and above caregiver reports, and vice versa, and at magnitudes that approximate typical correspondence levels between informants who observe adolescents in the same context (e.g., mother-father). Adolescent and peer confederate (but not caregiver) social anxiety reports predicted adolescents' state arousal in social interactions with unfamiliar peers
Karp et al. (2018)	A, Ca	Surveys, controlled observations	Surveys of adolescent functioning, self-reported arousal within interactions with unfamiliar peers	Adolescent and caregiver reports of evaluative fears (i.e., fears of positive and negative evaluation) display convergent validity as well as incremental and criterion-related validity; only adolescents' reports predicted adolescents' self-reported arousal within social interactions with unfamiliar peers

(continued)

Table 6.3 (continued)

Authors and publication year	Survey data sources	Instrumentation	Validity criteria	Summary of main findings
Keeley et al. (2018)	A, Ca	Surveys	Surveys of adolescent and family functioning	When assessing adolescent symptoms of attention-deficit/hyperactivity disorder (ADHD), adolescents' and caregivers' reports meaningfully vary in their links to validity indicators
Qasmieh et al. (2018)	A, Ca	Surveys, controlled observations	Surveys of adolescent functioning, self-reported arousal within interactions with unfamiliar peers	Adolescent and caregiver reports of safety behaviors display convergent validity as well as incremental and criterion-related validity; only adolescents' reports predicted adolescents' self-reported arousal within social interactions with unfamiliar peers
Byrne et al. (2019)	Ca	Surveys, controlled observations	Surveys of caregiver and family functioning, self-reported arousal within an impromptu speech task	This study supports the psychometric properties of the Emotion Reactivity Scale when administered in non-clinic assessments of adults
De Los Reyes et al. (2019d)	A, Ca	Surveys, controlled observations	Surveys of adolescent, caregiver, and family functioning; Ratings from trained independent observers	On both adolescent and caregiver versions of a measure of adolescent psychosocial impairments (i.e., the Work and Social Adjustment Scale for Youth [WSASY]), increased scores related to increased adolescent mental health concerns, adolescent-caregiver conflict, caregiver psychosocial dysfunction, and peer-related impairments. WSASY scores also distinguished adolescents who displayed co-occurring mental health concerns from those who did not and related to observed social skill deficits within social interactions with unfamiliar peers

(continued)

Table 6.3 (continued)

Authors and publication year	Survey data sources	Instrumentation	Validity criteria	Summary of main findings
Glenn et al. (2019)	A, Ca, PC	Surveys, controlled observations	Surveys of adolescent functioning, self-reported arousal within interactions with unfamiliar peers, ratings from trained independent observers	Observers' ratings were related to informants' survey reports of adolescent functioning. Observers' ratings distinguished adolescents on referral status and could distinguish adolescents on levels of social anxiety and social skills within specific kinds of social interactions with unfamiliar peers
Szollos et al. (2019)	A, Ca, PC	Surveys, controlled observations	Surveys of adolescent functioning, self-reported arousal within an impromptu speech task	Adolescents who displayed relatively high levels of both fears of negative evaluation and fears of positive evaluation (high FNE/FPE) tended to display poorer psychosocial functioning relative to adolescents who displayed other patterns of evaluative fears (i.e., low FNE/FPE, high on FNE but not FPE and vice versa). Based on adolescent-reported groups (but not caregiver-reported groups), high FNE/FPE adolescents displayed greater self-reported arousal during social interactions with unfamiliar peers, relative to the other groups.
Cannon et al. (2020)	A, Ca, PC	Surveys, controlled observations	Surveys of adolescent functioning, self-reported arousal within interactions with unfamiliar peers, ratings from trained independent observers	Leveraging experimental psychopathology and multi-modal assessment approaches, the Unfamiliar Peer Paradigm allows for understanding core components of social interactions with unfamiliar peers relevant to exposure-based therapy

(continued)

Table 6.3 (continued)

Authors and publication year	Survey data sources	Instrumentation	Validity criteria	Summary of main findings
Lipton et al. (2020)	Pa	Surveys, controlled observations	Surveys of caregiver functioning, self-reported arousal within an impromptu speech task, and tasks designed to communicate feedback about speech performance	On a task designed to simulate receipt of post-performance feedback (i.e., in reference to giving an impromptu speech), participants' self-reported fears of positive evaluation uniquely predicted arousal following receipt of positive feedback, whereas fears of negative evaluation uniquely predicted arousal following receipt of negative feedback. Relative to participants receiving positive feedback first, those receiving negative feedback first experienced elevated post-feedback arousal, followed by a steep decline in arousal post-positive feedback. Conversely, participants receiving positive feedback first experienced a buffer effect whereby arousal post-negative feedback remained low, relative to the arousal experienced post-negative feedback among those who received negative feedback first
Makol et al. (2020)	A, Ca, PC	Surveys, controlled observations	Surveys of adolescent functioning, ratings from trained independent observers	The Satellite Model's trait score incrementally predicted observed social anxiety (βs = 0.47–0.67) and referral status (odds ratios = 2.66–6.53) above and beyond individual informants' reports and a composite of these reports. The trait score predicted observed behavior at magnitudes well above those typically observed for individual informants' reports of internalizing psychopathology (i.e., rs = 0.01–0.15). Findings demonstrate the ability of the trait score to improve the prediction of clinical indices and potentially transform multi-informant assessment practices

(continued)

Table 6.3 (continued)

Authors and publication year	Survey data sources	Instrumentation	Validity criteria	Summary of main findings
Botkin et al. (2021)	A, Ca	Surveys, controlled observations	Surveys of adolescent functioning, ratings from trained independent observers	At the bivariate level, adolescents' FNE and FPE reports related to observed social anxiety and social skills, whereas caregivers' FPE reports related to observed social anxiety. Further, both informants' FPE reports demonstrated incremental validity in relation to observed social anxiety, relative to the other informant. Compared to their FNE reports, adolescents' PES reports displayed incremental validity in relation to observed social skills; the reverse was not true for adolescents' FNE reports
Rezeppa et al. (2021)	A, PC, UUO	Surveys, controlled observations	Surveys of adolescent functioning, self-reported arousal within interactions with unfamiliar peers, ratings from trained independent observers	Unfamiliar untrained observers' safety behavior reports (a) related to adolescents' safety behavior self-reports, (b) distinguished adolescents on clinically elevated social anxiety concerns, (c) related to trained independent observers' ratings of adolescent social skills within interactions with peer confederates, and (d) related to adolescents' self-reported arousal within these same interactions
Charamut et al. (2022)	A, Ca, UUO	Surveys, controlled observations	Surveys of adolescent and family functioning, self-reported arousal within interactions with unfamiliar peers, ratings from trained independent observers	Scores reflecting the Satellite Model's trait, context, and perspective components displayed distinct patterns of relations to a battery of criterion variables that varied in the context, perspective, and source of measurement. The Satellite Model instantiates situational specificity in measurement and facilitates unifying conceptual and measurement models of youth mental health

(continued)

Table 6.3 (continued)

Authors and publication year	Survey data sources	Instrumentation	Validity criteria	Summary of main findings
Greenberg and De Los Reyes (2022)	A, Pa,	Surveys, controlled observations	Surveys of adolescent functioning, ratings from trained independent observers	Adolescents with co-occurring social anxiety and ADHD symptoms displayed significantly lower social skills, relative to all other groups (i.e., low social anxiety and ADHD, high social anxiety and low ADHD, and vice versa)
Okuno et al. (2022)	A, Ca, PC, UUO	Surveys, controlled observations	Surveys of adolescent functioning, ratings from trained independent observers	Relative to other adolescents in the sample, adolescents high on both safety behaviors and social anxiety displayed greater psychosocial impairments and evaluative fears and observed social skill deficits within social interactions with unfamiliar peers
Bellamy et al. (2023)	Ca	Surveys, controlled observations	Surveys of adolescent and family functioning, self-reported arousal within interactions with unfamiliar peers, ratings from trained independent observers	Findings supported the incremental validity of scores taken from caregivers' reports of adolescent psychopathy and across multiple criterion variables, including (a) an established survey measure of caregiver-adolescent conflict and (b) trained independent observers' ratings of adolescents' behavioral reactions to laboratory-controlled tasks designed to simulate social interactions with unfamiliar peers
Follet et al. (2023)	A, Ca, PC, UUO	Surveys, controlled observations	Surveys of adolescent functioning, ratings from trained independent observers	Caregivers' reports performed best when distinguishing adolescents on referral status and predicting survey-reported social anxiety, whereas only UUOs' reports predicted independent observers' social skill ratings. These findings inform the strategic selection of informants for assessing impairments that commonly prompt the need for adolescents to access mental health services for social anxiety

(continued)

Table 6.3 (continued)

Authors and publication year	Survey data sources	Instrumentation	Validity criteria	Summary of main findings
Sangraula and De Los Reyes (2024)	Ca	Surveys	Surveys of caregiver, adolescent, and family functioning	This study supports the psychometric properties of the Quality of Life Enjoyment and Satisfaction Questionnaire-Short Form when administered in non-clinic assessments of adults
Keeley et al. (2024)	A, Ca	Surveys, controlled observations	Surveys of family functioning, ratings from trained independent observers	Discrepancies between caregiver and adolescent survey reports of parental monitoring predict adolescents' anxiety within interactions with unfamiliar peers
Racz et al. (2024)	A, Ca	Surveys, controlled observations	Surveys of adolescent and caregiver functioning, self-reported arousal within interactions with unfamiliar peers, self-reported arousal within an impromptu speech task	Subfactors of safety behaviors exist (i.e., avoidance and impression management), and these factors differentially predict fears of negative and positive evaluation
Bellamy et al. (2024)	A, Ca	Surveys, controlled observations	Surveys of adolescent and family functioning, self-reported arousal at rest within a controlled laboratory setting	Adolescents' resting arousal moderates links between parental monitoring and adolescent psychopathy, with these moderating effects varying by psychopathy domain and the informants reporting about parental monitoring and adolescent psychopathy

Note: *A* adolescent, *Ca* caregiver, *PC* peer confederate, *UUO* unfamiliar untrained observer. (Adapted from the accepted manuscript version of De Los Reyes, 2024)

adolescent participants within the behavioral tasks described below. They also completed survey measures about adolescent social anxiety, using the parallel format that parents and adolescents used to make their own reports about adolescent social anxiety. Following the study, we provided feedback to clinic-referred families on their adolescent's mental health concerns and referrals for mental health services.

To be eligible for the study, we required dyads to (a) be fluent in English, (b) understand the consenting and interview process, (c) have a 14–15-year-old adolescent currently living in the home with the caregiver completing the study, and (d) have an adolescent whom the caregiver did not report as having a history of learning or developmental disabilities. The total sample included 134 caregiver-adolescent dyads (45 clinic-referred, 89 community control). Adolescents were 14 or 15 years old ($M_{age} = 14.49$, $SD = 0.50$); 89 adolescents identified as female, and 45 identified as male. Based on parent reports, adolescents' race/ethnicity included African American/Black (53.0%), Caucasian/European American/White (33.6%), Hispanic/Spanish/Latino/a (10.4%), Asian American/Asian (5.2%), American Indian (0.7%), or other (e.g., Caribbean; 7.5%). Race/ethnicity values total above 100% given that caregivers could select multiple racial/ethnic categories. Caregivers included the adolescent's biological mother or father (95.5%), adoptive mother or father (2.2%), or another caregiver (2.2%). Caregivers reported household income using a scale with ten categories that varied by $100 increments (i.e., less than $100 per week through $901 or more per week). Based on this scale, 26.1% of families had a weekly household income of $500 or less, 22.4% had a weekly household income between $501 and $900, and 51.5% had a weekly household income of $901 or more per week.

In all study analyses, we pooled participants across recruitment strategies (i.e., clinic-referred, community control). By design, we recruited community-control adolescents in larger numbers than clinic-referred adolescents. We selected this approach given that it mimics displays of dimensionally varying social anxiety in the general population and is consistent with dimensional models of psychopathology (Casey et al., 2014). We also used this recruitment strategy given that dimensional approaches offer greater reliability and validity relative to categorical approaches (Markon et al., 2011). Further, this approach is consistent with prior studies leveraging similar recruitment strategies, most notably the Tracking Adolescents' Individual Lives Survey (e.g., TRAILS; Bouma et al., 2009).

As with TRAILS, our recruitment strategies did not introduce confounds when interpreting our findings. Our two recruitment strategies did not produce adolescents who varied on the demographic characteristics reported previously. To demonstrate this, we conducted analyses to determine whether participants across the two strategies differed on key demographic characteristics including adolescent age, adolescent gender, adolescent racial/ethnic background, family income, caregiver relation to the adolescent, and caregiver marital status. Given the exploratory nature of these tests, we applied a Bonferroni correction (i.e., 11 tests and thus a corrected p-value cutoff of 0.0045). These analyses revealed no significant demographic differences between participants recruited via the two strategies.

As an additional justification of our pooled sampling approach, prior work in this same sample has followed recommendations for probing patterns of relations among variables of interest (Hassler & Thadewald, 2003; Powers & Powers, 2015). Specifically, in two separate investigations (Glenn et al., 2019; Keeley et al., 2024), our team has inspected the range of correlations between our survey reports of various behavioral domains (e.g., adolescent and family functioning) and independent observers' ratings of adolescent behavior (i.e., our validity criteria for Study 2), relative to the range of partial correlations that controlled for method of recruitment (i.e., clinic-referred, community control). In essence, these tests addressed the key issue of whether our approach involved pooling heterogeneous samples that should have, instead, been examined separately. In our prior work, we have not observed differences in correlations that were substantial enough to rule out taking a pooled sample approach to address our aims. Further, the tests conducted by Glenn et al. (2019) among survey reports and observed behavior leveraged the same instruments used for Study 2. As such, we took a pooled sampling approach to address the aims of Study 2.

6.2.2 *Survey Measures*

Caregivers completed a demographic questionnaire. Caregivers, adolescents, and peer confederates completed measures to assess the adolescent's social anxiety, and caregivers completed a measure to assess their own depressive symptoms. For measures completed by more than one informant, parallel survey items were used, with only minor modifications made to fit each informant's perspective (i.e., "My child" for caregiver measures, "I" for adolescent measures, "The participant" for peer confederates). Caregivers and adolescents completed measures before the adolescent's participation in social interaction tasks. Peer confederates completed survey measures following their interactions with adolescents in these tasks.

6.2.2.1 Social Phobia Scale (SPS; Mattick & Clarke, 1998)

Caregivers, adolescents, and peer confederates completed the 20-item SPS. To reduce the number of indicators when using the SPS within the Trifactor Models, we used a six-item short form (i.e., SPS-6; Peters et al., 2012). The SPS assesses adolescents' fears of being scrutinized by others during routine activities (example item, "I/My child/The participant is/am worried about shaking or trembling when watched by other people."). Informants rated items on a Likert scale ranging from 0 (*Not at all characteristic or true of me/my child/the participant*) to 4 (*Extremely characteristic or true of me/my child/the participant*). The 20-item SPS exhibits strong validity, differentiates individuals on diagnostic status, and is sensitive to treatment response (Mattick & Clarke, 1998; Deros et al., 2018). Similarly, the SPS-6 demonstrates adequate internal consistency and convergent validity, differentiates individuals with and without social anxiety concerns, and is sensitive to treatment response (Carleton et al., 2014; Fergus et al., 2014; Peters et al., 2012). Adolescent (SPS $\alpha = 0.92$; SPS-6 $\alpha = 0.87$), caregiver (SPS $\alpha = 0.94$; SPS-6 $\alpha = 0.89$), and peer confederates' reports (SPS $\alpha = 0.96$; SPS-6 $\alpha = 0.90$) on the SPS and SPS-6 exhibited good-to-excellent internal consistency and were highly correlated ($rs = 0.95$–0.96, $ps < 0.001$). We used informants' SPS-6 reports in the Trifactor Models. In addition, we used informants' SPS reports in incremental validity analyses comparing the performance of the Satellite Model *Trait* score relative to individual informants' reports and the composite score when predicting independent criterion variables.

6.2.2.2 Social Interaction Anxiety Scale (SIAS; Mattick & Clarke, 1998)

Informants completed the 20-item SIAS, which is a measure for assessing social anxiety concerns that adolescents may experience during social interactions (example item, "I/my child/the participant has difficulty talking with other people."). Informants rated items on a Likert scale ranging from 0 (*Not at all characteristic or true of me/my child/the participant*) to 4 (*Extremely characteristic or true of me/my child/the participant*). Informants' reports on the SIAS display convergent validity and distinguish adolescents on referral status (Deros et al., 2018; Glenn et al., 2019). Adolescent ($\alpha = 0.94$), caregiver ($\alpha = 0.95$), and peer confederate reports ($\alpha = 0.96$) exhibited excellent internal consistency. We used informants' SIAS reports in the Satellite Model. In addition, we used informants' SIAS reports in incremental validity analyses comparing the performance of the Trifactor Model *Common Factor* score relative to individual informants' reports and the composite score when predicting independent criterion variables.

6.2.2.3 Social Phobia and Anxiety Inventory for Children (SPAIC; Beidel et al., 1995)

Caregivers and adolescents completed the 26-item SPAIC, which is one of the most widely used youth social anxiety measures. The SPAIC requires informants to endorse how often the adolescent feels nervous or scared when in various social scenarios (e.g., meeting new peers). Several items include "sub-items" that require informants to rate the adolescent's social anxiety with different interaction partners (e.g., "boys or girls his/her age that he/she knows" vs. "boys or girls his/her age that he/she doesn't know"). These sub-items are averaged at the item level to create a composite score. Caregivers and adolescents rated items using a Likert scale ranging from 0 (*never*) to 2 (*always*). Caregiver and adolescent reports on the SPAIC display strong construct and convergent validity, relate to independent observers' ratings of anxiety and social skills, differentiate adolescents on referral status, and are sensitive to treatment response (Beidel et al., 1995, 2000a, b). Adolescent ($\alpha = 0.95$) and caregiver reports ($\alpha = 0.96$) exhibited excellent internal consistency. We used adolescents' and caregivers' SPAIC reports in incremental validity analyses comparing the performance of the Trifactor Model *Common Factor* and Satellite Model *Trait* scores to individual informants' reports when predicting independent criterion variables.

6.2.2.4 Beck Depression Inventory-II (BDI-II; Beck et al., 1996)

Caregivers completed a modified version of the BDI-II, a 21-item measure commonly used to screen for depression. Caregivers rated their own depressive symptoms using a three-point scale on which higher scores indicated higher levels of depressive symptoms. Based on the study's protocol, we did not administer items 9 and 21 of the BDI-II (see Rausch et al., 2017). For this reason, we prorated items 9 and 21 by calculating a mean item score for each participant and including a prorated item score for items 9 and 21. The BDI-II demonstrates strong psychometric properties across studies, including strong reliability, strong criterion-related validity, and good sensitivity and specificity when predicting depression diagnosis (Wang & Gorenstein, 2013). Caregiver reports on the BDI-II exhibited excellent internal consistency ($\alpha = 0.92$). We entered caregiver BDI-II reports as an informant-level predictor in Trifactor Models that included caregiver reports.

6.2.3 Unfamiliar Peer Paradigm and Independent Observer Ratings

Following completion of self-report measures, adolescents participated in the Unfamiliar Peer Paradigm (Fig. 6.1; Cannon et al., 2020)—a series of counterbalanced social interaction tasks with peer confederates that vary in terms of structure and content (e.g., Curran et al., 2020; Beidel et al., 2000a, 2010). Based on adolescents' reactions to these tasks, we obtained independent observers' ratings of

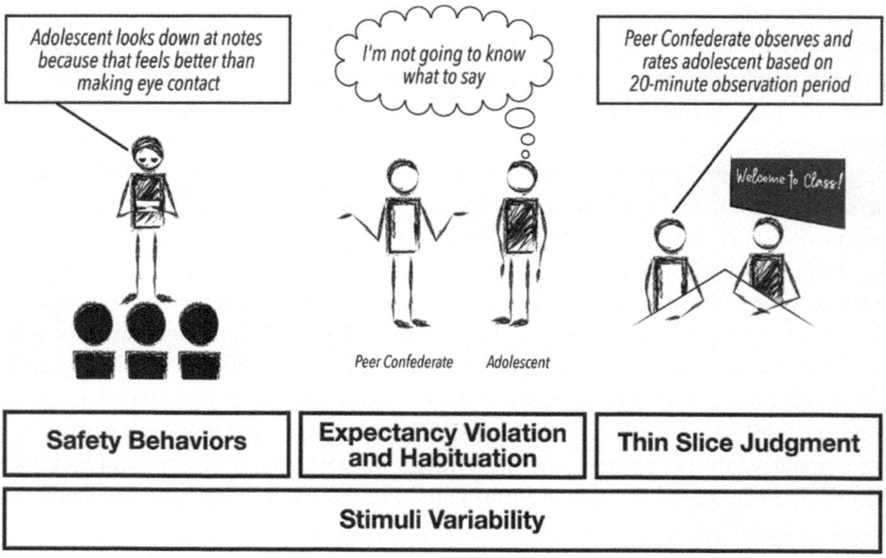

Fig. 6.1 The conceptual and empirical foundations of the Unfamiliar Peer Paradigm. *Note*: The Unfamiliar Peer Paradigm's origins lie in research and theory in clinical psychology on mechanisms of change in exposure-based therapies, namely, work on clients' use of safety behaviors during therapeutic exposures, the need to consider stimuli variability or the degree to which exposures vary on key elements of anxiety-provoking situations, and the importance of expectancy violation and habituation processes in therapy. The paradigm's origins also lie in research and theory in personality and social psychology on thin-slice judgments or the ability to gather data about adolescent social anxiety based on the small "samples" of behavior displayed during tasks within the paradigm. (Reproduced from the accepted manuscript version of Cannon et al., 2020)

adolescent social anxiety using a validated behavioral coding scheme developed by Beidel and colleagues (Beidel et al., 2000a, 2010) and validated within this sample (Glenn et al., 2019). Along with adolescents' referral status (i.e., clinic-referred vs. community control), we used independent observers' ratings of adolescent social anxiety as validity criteria.

6.2.3.1 Descriptions of Tasks in Unfamiliar Peer Paradigm

Following the completion of self-report measures, adolescents participated in a series of counterbalanced social interaction tasks with peer confederates. These tasks were developed in prior work with children, adolescents, and adults (e.g., Beidel et al., 2000a, 2010) and took approximately 20 min to complete. Tasks included the Unstructured Conversation Task (UCT; adapted from Beidel et al., 2010), Simulated Social Interaction Test (SSIT; adapted from Curran et al., 2020; Beidel et al., 2000a), and Impromptu Speech Task (IST; adapted from Beidel et al., 2010). In each task, adolescents interacted with research assistants trained to pose as adolescents (i.e., peer confederates). We masked peer confederates to adolescents' referral status and clinical information and ensured they had no prior interaction with adolescents or their caregivers prior to beginning the task. In all one-on-one social interactions, we paired adolescents with a peer confederate matched to the gender identity reported by families on our demographic survey.

In the UCT, adolescents participated in an unstructured 3-min role-play with a peer confederate. We provided the following instructions to adolescents: "*Pretend that you are at a new school and don't know anyone.*" We trained peer confederates to respond neutrally and allow the adolescent to drive the conversation. In the SSIT, adolescents participated in a series of five one-to-three-minute role-playing scenes (e.g., offering/accepting assistance, responding to inappropriate behavior) with a peer confederate. In each role-play, adolescents were provided two opportunities to speak, and peer confederates were trained to provide two scripted responses. In the IST, adolescents participated in a speech task in which they delivered a speech to a small audience about topics infrequently discussed by adolescents (e.g., politics, public health). The audience included a task administrator and two trained peer confederates with whom the adolescent had no prior contact. We provided adolescents 3 min to prepare their speech and 10 min to complete their speech. Following a minimum period of 3 min into the speech, we permitted adolescents to terminate the speech if they wished to do so. We video-recorded social interaction tasks from two angles to allow for the coding of adolescent behavior.

6.2.3.2 Behavioral Ratings Based on Unfamiliar Peer Paradigm

To obtain independent observers' ratings of adolescent social anxiety in social interaction tasks, we used a validated behavioral coding scheme developed by Beidel and colleagues (Beidel et al., 2000a, 2010). We ensured that independent observers had no prior interactions with adolescents in social interaction tasks and were masked to adolescents' referral status and clinical information. Two independent observers provided macro-level ratings of adolescent social anxiety on a five-point scale ranging from 1 (*animated*) to 5 (*severe anxiety*). Independent observers made a total of seven ratings (i.e., one UCT rating, five SSIT ratings, one IST rating), and these ratings were used to compute a social anxiety composite. Inter-rater reliability for the two independent observers' ratings of social anxiety was in the good range (average $ICC = 0.76$). This coding scheme has been used extensively in prior work seeking to understand adolescent behavior when interacting with unfamiliar peers (e.g., Bellamy et al., 2023; Botkin et al., 2021; Cannon et al., 2020; Charamut et al., 2022; Follet et al., 2023; Glenn et al., 2019; Greenberg & De Los Reyes, 2022; Keeley et al., 2024; Makol et al., 2020; Okuno et al., 2022; Rezeppa et al., 2021).

6.3 Concluding Comments

This chapter described key features of validity criteria used by scholars in youth development and linked these features to the notion of situational specificity. These crucial elements of work in youth development call for context-sensitive validity criteria. When coupled with the use of structurally different informants, these elements play consequential roles in the design of measurement validation studies, particularly those focused on probing the criterion-related validity of scores taken from instruments. Along these lines, we described the design of Study 2—a measurement validation study designed using the principles that underlie CONTEXT. In Chap. 7, we report the analytic plan and findings from Study 2.

References

Achenbach, T. M., McConaughy, S. H., & Howell, C. T. (1987). Child/adolescent behavioral and emotional problems: Implications of cross-informant correlations for situational specificity. *Psychological Bulletin, 101*(2), 213–232. https://psycnet.apa.org/doi/10.1037/0033-2909.101.2.213

Alfano, C. A., & Beidel, D. C. (2011). *Social anxiety in adolescents and young adults: Translating developmental science into practice*. American Psychological Association.

Bandura, A. (1977). *Social learning theory*. Prentice-Hall.

Beale, A., Keeley, L. M., Okuno, H., Szollos, S., Rausch, E., Makol, B. A., Augenstein, T. M., Lipton, M. F., Racz, S. J., & De Los Reyes, A. (2018). Efficient screening for impairments in peer functioning among mid-to-late adolescents receiving clinical assessments for social anxiety. *Child and Youth Care Forum, 47*(5), 613–631. https://doi.org/10.1007/s10566-018-9458-x

Beck, A. T. (1993). Cognitive therapy: Past, present, and future. *Journal of Consulting and Clinical Psychology, 61*(2), 194–198. https://doi.org/10.1037/0022-006X.61.2.194

Beck, A. T., Steer, R. A., & Brown, G. K. (1996). *Beck depression inventory–Second edition manual*. The Psychological Corporation.

Beidel, D. C., Turner, S. M., Jacob, R. G., & Cooley, M. R. (1989). Assessment of social phobia: Reliability of an impromptu speech task. *Journal of Anxiety Disorders, 3*(3), 149–158. https://doi.org/10.1016/0887-6185(89)90009-1

Beidel, D. C., Turner, S. M., & Morris, T. L. (1995). A new inventory to assess childhood social anxiety and phobia: The Social Phobia and Anxiety Inventory for Children. *Psychological Assessment, 7*(1), 73–79. https://doi.org/10.1037/1040-3590.7.1.73

Beidel, D. S., Turner, S. M., Hamlin, K., & Morris, T. L. (2000a). The Social Phobia and Anxiety Inventory for Children (SPAI-C): External and discriminative validity. *Behavior Therapy, 31*(1), 75–87. https://psycnet.apa.org/doi/10.1016/S0005-7894(00)80005-2

Beidel, D. C., Turner, S. M., & Morris, T. L. (2000b). Behavioral treatment of childhood social phobia. *Journal of Consulting and Clinical Psychology, 68*(6), 1072–1080. https://psycnet.apa.org/doi/10.1037/0022-006X.68.6.1072

Beidel, D. C., Rao, P. A., Scharfstein, L., Wong, N., & Alfano, C. A. (2010). Social skills and social phobia: An investigation of DSM-IV subtypes. *Behaviour Research and Therapy, 48*(10), 992–1001. https://psycnet.apa.org/doi/10.1016/j.brat.2010.06.005

Bellamy, N., Salekin, R. T., Makol, B. A., Augenstein, T. M., & De Los Reyes, A. (2023). The Proposed Specifiers for Conduct Disorder—Parent (PSCD-P): Convergent validity, incremental validity, and reactions to unfamiliar peer confederates. *Research on Child and Adolescent Psychopathology., 51*(8), 1097–1113. https://doi.org/10.1007/s10802-023-01056-x

Bellamy, N., Salekin, R. T., Racz, S. J., & De Los Reyes, A. (2024). A multi-dimensional, multi-informant examination of adolescent psychopathy and its links to parental monitoring: The moderating role of resting arousal. *Prevention Science*. Advance online publication. https://doi.org/10.1007/s11121-024-01753-z

Benner, G. J., Strycker, L. A., Ralston, N. C., Michael, E., Jolivette, K., Baylin, A., & Zeng, S. (2022). Promoting engagement of US elementary students with emotional and behavioral disorders: evidence of efficacy of the Classroom Reset program. *International Journal of Educational Research Open, 3*, 100122. https://doi.org/10.1016/j.ijedro.2022.100122

Botkin, T., Racz, S. J., Makol, B. A., & De Los Reyes, A. (2021). Multi-informant assessments of adolescents' fears of negative and positive evaluation: Criterion-related and incremental validity in relation to observed behavior. *Journal of Psychopathology and Behavioral Assessment, 43*(1), 58–69. https://doi.org/10.1007/s10862-020-09855-y

Bouma, E. M., Riese, H., Ormel, J., Verhulst, F. C., & Oldehinkel, A. J. (2009). Adolescents' cortisol responses to awakening and social stress; effects of gender, menstrual phase and oral contraceptives. The TRAILS study. *Psychoneuroendocrinology, 34*(6), 884–893. https://doi.org/10.1016/j.psyneuen.2009.01.003

Bousha, D. M., & Twentyman, C. T. (1984). Mother–child interactional style in abuse, neglect, and control groups: Naturalistic observations in the home. *Journal of Abnormal Psychology, 93*(1), 106–114. https://doi.org/10.1037/0021-843X.93.1.106

Byrne, S., Makol, B. A., Keeley, L. M., & De Los Reyes, A. (2019). Psychometric properties of the Emotion Reactivity Scale in community screening assessments. *Journal of Psychopathology and Behavioral Assessment, 41*(4), 730–740. https://doi.org/10.1007/s10862-019-09749-8

Cannon, C. J., Makol, B. A., Keeley, L. M., Qasmieh, N., Okuno, H., Racz, S. J., & De Los Reyes, A. (2020). A paradigm for understanding adolescent social anxiety with unfamiliar peers: Conceptual foundations and directions for future research. *Clinical Child and Family Psychology Review, 23*(3), 338–364. https://doi.org/10.1007/s10567-020-00314-4

Carleton, R. N., Thibodeau, M. A., Weeks, J. W., Teale Sapach, M. J. N., McEvoy, P. M., Horswill, S. C., & Heimberg, R. G. (2014). Comparing short forms of the Social Interaction Anxiety Scale and the Social Phobia Scale. *Psychological Assessment, 26*(4), 1116–1126. https://psycnet.apa.org/doi/10.1037/a0037063

Casey, B. J., Oliveri, M. E., & Insel, T. (2014). A neurodevelopmental perspective on the research domain criteria (RDoC) framework. *Biological Psychiatry, 76*(5), 350–353. https://doi.org/10.1016/j.biopsych.2014.01.006

Charamut, N. R., Racz, S. J., Wang, M., & De Los Reyes, A. (2022). Integrating multi-informant reports of youth mental health: A construct validation test of Kraemer and Colleagues' (2003) Satellite Model. *Frontiers in Psychology, 13*, 911629. https://doi.org/10.3389/fpsyg.2022.911629

Curran, P. J., Georgeson, A. R., Bauer, D. J., & Hussong, A. M. (2020). Psychometric models for scoring multiple reporter assessments: Applications to integrative data analysis in prevention science and beyond. *International Journal of Behavioral Development, 45*(1), 40–50. https://doi.org/10.1177/0165025419896620

Daley, D., Sonuga-Barke, E. J. S., & Thompson, M. (2003). Assessing expressed emotion in mothers of preschool AD/HD children: Psychometric properties of a modified speech sample. *British Journal of Clinical Psychology, 42*(1), 53–67. https://doi.org/10.1348/014466503762842011

d'Apice, K., Latham, R. M., & von Stumm, S. (2019). A naturalistic home observational approach to children's language, cognition, and behavior. *Developmental Psychology, 55*(7), 1414–1427. https://doi.org/10.1037/dev0000733

De Los Reyes, A. (2024). *Discrepant results in mental health research: What they mean, why they matter, and how they inform scientific practices*. Oxford University Press.

De Los Reyes, A., & Aldao, A. (2015). Introduction to the special issue. Toward implementing physiological measures in clinical child and adolescent assessments. *Journal of Clinical Child and Adolescent Psychology, 44*(2), 221–237. https://doi.org/10.1080/15374416.2014.891227

De Los Reyes, A., Augenstein, T. M., & Aldao, A. (2017a). Assessment issues in child and adolescent psychotherapy. In J. R. Weisz & A. E. Kazdin (Eds.), *Evidence-based psychotherapies for children and adolescents* (3rd ed., pp. 537–554). Guilford.

De Los Reyes, A., Aldao, A., Qasmieh, N., Dunn, E. J., Lipton, M. F., Hartman, C., Dougherty, L. R., Youngstrom, E. A., & Lerner, M. D. (2017b). Graphical representations of adolescents' psychophysiological reactivity to social stressor tasks: Reliability and validity of the Chernoff Face approach and person-centered profiles for clinical use. *Psychological Assessment, 29*(4), 422–434. https://doi.org/10.1037/pas0000354

De Los Reyes, A., Ohannessian, C. M., & Racz, S. J. (2019a). Discrepancies between adolescent and parent reports about family relationships. *Child Development Perspectives, 13*(1), 53–58. https://doi.org/10.1111/cdep.12306

De Los Reyes, A., Lerner, M. D., Keeley, L. M., Weber, R. J., Drabick, D. A., Rabinowitz, J., & Goodman, K. L. (2019b). Improving interpretability of subjective assessments about psychological phenomena: a review and cross-cultural meta-analysis. *Review of General Psychology, 23*(3), 293–319. https://doi.org/10.1177/1089268019837645

De Los Reyes, A., Cook, C. R., Gresham, F. M., Makol, B. A., & Wang, M. (2019c). Informant discrepancies in assessments of psychosocial functioning in school-based services and research: Review and directions for future research. *Journal of School Psychology, 74*, 74–89. https://doi.org/10.1016/j.jsp.2019.05.005

De Los Reyes, A., Makol, B. A., Racz, S. J., Youngstrom, E. A., Lerner, M. D., & Keeley, L. M. (2019d). The Work and Social Adjustment Scale for Youth: A measure for assessing youth psychosocial impairment regardless of mental health status. *Journal of Child and Family Studies, 28*(1), 1–16. https://doi.org/10.1007/s10826-018-1238-6

De Los Reyes, A., Talbott, E., Power, T., Michel, J., Cook, C. R., Racz, S. J., & Fitzpatrick, O. (2022a). The Needs-to-Goals Gap: How informant discrepancies in youth mental health assessments impact service delivery. *Clinical Psychology Review, 92*, Article 102114. https://doi.org/10.1016/j.cpr.2021.102114

De Los Reyes, A., Tyrell, F. A., Watts, A. L., & Asmundson, G. J. G. (2022b). Conceptual, methodological, and measurement factors that disqualify use of measurement invariance techniques to detect informant discrepancies in youth mental health assessments. *Frontiers in Psychology, 13*, Article 931296. https://doi.org/10.3389/fpsyg.2022.931296

De Los Reyes, A., Cook, C. R., Sullivan, M., Morrell, N., Hamlin, C., Wang, M., Gresham, F. M., Makol, B. A., Keeley, L. M., & Qasmieh, N. (2022c). The Work and Social Adjustment Scale for Youth: Psychometric properties of the teacher version and evidence of contextual variability in psychosocial impairments. *Psychological Assessment, 34*(8), 777–790. https://doi.org/10.1037/pas0001139

De Los Reyes, A., Wang, M., Lerner, M. D., Makol, B. A., Fitzpatrick, O., & Weisz, J. R. (2023a). The Operations Triad Model and youth mental health assessments: Catalyzing a paradigm shift in measurement validation. *Journal of Clinical Child and Adolescent Psychology, 52*(1), 19–54. https://doi.org/10.1080/15374416.2022.2111684

De Los Reyes, A., Epkins, C. C., Asmundson, G. J. G., Augenstein, T. M., Becker, K. D., Becker, S. P., Bonadio, F. T., Borelli, J. L., Boyd, R. C., Bradshaw, C. P., Burns, G. L., Casale, G., Causadias, J. M., Cha, C. B., Chorpita, B. F., Cohen, J. R., Comer, J. S., Crowell, S. E., Dirks, M. A., et al. (2023b). Editorial statement about *JCCAP*'s 2023 special issue on informant discrepancies in youth mental health assessments: Observations, guidelines, and future directions grounded in 60 years of research. *Journal of Clinical Child and Adolescent Psychology, 52*(1), 147–158. https://doi.org/10.1080/15374416.2022.2158842

Deros, D. E., Racz, S. J., Lipton, M. F., Augenstein, T. M., Karp, J. N., Keeley, L. M., et al. (2018). Multi-informant assessments of adolescent social anxiety: Adding clarity by leveraging reports from unfamiliar peer confederates. *Behavior Therapy, 49*(1), 84–98. https://doi.org/10.1016/j.beth.2017.05.001

DeWall, C., MacDonald, G., Webster, G. D., Masten, C. L., Baumeister, R. F., Powell, C., Combs, D., Schurtz, D. R., Stillman, T. F., Tice, D. M., & Eisenberger, N. I. (2010). Acetaminophen reduces social pain: Behavioral and neural evidence. *Psychological Science, 21*(7), 931–937. https://doi.org/10.1177/0956797610374741

Dickerson, S. S., & Kemeny, M. E. (2004). Acute stressors and cortisol responses: A theoretical integration and synthesis of laboratory research. *Psychological Bulletin, 130*(3), 355–391. https://doi.org/10.1037/0033-2909.130.3.355

Donenberg, G. R., & Weisz, J. R. (1997). Experimental task and speaker effects on parent–child interactions of aggressive and depressed/anxious children. *Journal of Abnormal Child Psychology, 25*(5), 367–387. https://doi.org/10.1023/A:1025733023979

Fanger, S. M., Frankel, L. A., & Hazen, N. (2012). Peer exclusion in preschool children's play: Naturalistic observations in a playground setting. *Merrill-Palmer Quarterly, 58*(2), 224–254. https://doi.org/10.1353/mpq.2012.0007

Fergus, T. A., Valentiner, D. P., Kim, H. S., & McGrath, P. B. (2014). The Social Interaction Anxiety Scale (SIAS) and the Social Phobia Scale (SPS): A comparison of two short-form versions. *Psychological Assessment, 26*(4), 1281–1291. https://doi.org/10.1037/a0037313

Follet, L., Okuno, H., & De Los Reyes, A. (2023). Assessing peer-related impairments linked to adolescent social anxiety: Strategic selection of informants optimizes prediction of clinically relevant domains. *Behavior Therapy, 54*(1), 29–42. https://doi.org/10.1016/j.beth.2022.06.010

Garb, H. N. (2003). Incremental validity and the assessment of psychopathology in adults. *Psychological Assessment, 15*(4), 508–520. https://doi.org/10.1037/1040-3590.15.4.508

Glenn, L. E., Keeley, L. M., Szollos, S., Okuno, H., Wang, X., Rausch, E., Deros, D. E., Karp, J. N., Qasmieh, N., Makol, B. A., Augenstein, T. M., Lipton, M. F., Racz, S. J., Scharfstein, L., Beidel, D. C., & De Los Reyes, A. (2019). Trained observers' ratings of adolescents' social anxiety and social skills within controlled, cross-contextual social interactions with unfamiliar peer confederates. *Journal of Psychopathology and Behavioral Assessment, 41*(1), 1–15. https://doi.org/10.1007/s10862-018-9676-4

Greenberg, A., & De Los Reyes, A. (2022). When adolescents experience co-occurring social anxiety and ADHD symptoms: Links with social skills when interacting with unfamiliar peer confederates. *Behavior Therapy, 53*(6), 1109–1121. https://doi.org/10.1016/j.beth.2022.04.011

Gresham, F. M., Elliott, S. N., Cook, C. R., Vance, M. J., & Kettler, R. (2010). Cross-informant agreement for ratings for social skill and problem behavior ratings: An investigation of the Social Skills Improvement System—Rating Scales. *Psychological Assessment, 22*(1), 157–166. https://doi.org/10.1037/a0018124

Groth-Marnat, G., & Wright, A. J. (2016). *Handbook of psychological assessment* (6th ed.). Wiley.

Gunnar, M. R., Talge, N. M., & Herrera, A. (2009). Stressor paradigms in developmental studies: What does and does not work to produce mean increases in salivary cortisol. *Psychoneuroendocrinology, 34*(7), 953–967. https://doi.org/10.1016/j.psyneuen.2009.02.010

Hassler, U., & Thadewald, T. (2003). Nonsensical and biased correlation due to pooling heterogeneous samples. *The Statistician, 52*(3), 367–379. Retrieved from http://www.jstor.org/stable/4128210

Hooley, J. M., & Parker, H. A. (2006). Measuring expressed emotion: An evaluation of the shortcuts. *Journal of Family Psychology, 20*(3), 386–396. https://doi.org/10.1037/0893-3200.20.3.386

Hunsley, J., & Meyer, G. J. (2003). The incremental validity of psychological testing and assessment: Conceptual, methodological, and statistical issues. *Psychological Assessment, 15*(4), 446–455. https://doi.org/10.1037/1040-3590.15.4.446

Jeon, E. H., & Yamashito, J. (2014). L2 reading comprehension and its correlates: A meta-analysis. *Language Learning, 64*(1), 160–212. https://doi.org/10.1111/lang.12034

Karp, J. N., Makol, B. A., Keeley, L. M., Qasmieh, N., Deros, D. E., Weeks, J. W., Racz, S. J., Lipton, M. F., Augenstein, T. M., & De Los Reyes, A. (2018). Convergent, incremental, and criterion-related validity of multi-informant assessments of adolescents' fears of negative and positive evaluation. *Clinical Psychology and Psychotherapy, 25*(2), 217–230. https://doi.org/10.1002/cpp.2156

Keeley, L. M., Makol, B. A., Qasmieh, N., Deros, D. E., Karp, J. N., Lipton, M. F., Augenstein, T. M., Truong, M. L., Racz, S. J., & De Los Reyes, A. (2018). Validity of adolescent and parent reports on the Six-Item ADHD Self-Report Scale (ASRS-6) in clinical assessments of adolescent social anxiety. *Journal of Child and Family Studies, 27*(4), 1041–1053. https://doi.org/10.1007/s10826-017-0950-y

Keeley, L. M., Laird, R. D., Qasmieh, N., Racz, S. J., Ohannessian, C. M., & De Los Reyes, A. (2024). When parents and adolescents make discrepant reports about parental monitoring: Links to adolescent anxiety when interacting with unfamiliar peers. *Journal of Psychopathology and Behavioral Assessment, 46*(2), 343–356. https://doi.org/10.1007/s10862-024-10132-5

Kiecolt-Glaser, J. K., Loving, T. J., Stowell, J. R., Malarkey, W. B., Lemeshow, S., Dickinson, S. L., & Glaser, R. (2005). Hostile marital interactions, proinflammatory cytokine production, and wound healing. *Archives of General Psychiatry, 62*(12), 1377–1384. https://doi.org/10.1001/archpsyc.62.12.1377

Lakind, D., Bradley, W. J., Patel, A., Chorpita, B. F., & Becker, K. D. (2022). A multidimensional examination of the measurement of treatment engagement: Implications for children's mental health services and research. *Journal of Clinical Child and Adolescent Psychology, 51*(4), 453–468. https://doi.org/10.1080/15374416.2021.1941057

Lin, X., Peng, P., & Zeng, J. (2021). Understanding the relation between mathematics vocabulary and mathematics performance: A Meta-analysis. *The Elementary School Journal, 121*(3), 504–540. https://doi.org/10.1086/712504

Lipton, M. F., Qasmieh, N., Racz, S. J., Weeks, J. W., & De Los Reyes, A. (2020). The Fears of Evaluation about Performance (FEAP) task: Inducing anxiety-related responses to direct exposure to negative and positive evaluations. *Behavior Therapy, 51*(6), 843–855. https://doi.org/10.1016/j.beth.2020.01.004

Makol, B. A., De Los Reyes, A., Ostrander, R., & Reynolds, E. K. (2019). Parent-youth divergence (and convergence) in reports of youth internalizing problems in psychiatric inpatient care. *Journal of Abnormal Child Psychology, 47*(10), 1677–1689. https://doi.org/10.1007/s10802-019-00540-7

Makol, B. A., Youngstrom, E. A., Racz, S. J., Qasmieh, N., Glenn, L. E., & De Los Reyes, A. (2020). Integrating multiple informants' reports: How conceptual and measurement models may address long-standing problems in clinical decision-making. *Clinical Psychological Science, 8*(6), 953–970. https://doi.org/10.1177/2167702620924439

Marci, C. D., Ham, J., Moran, E., & Orr, S. P. (2007). Physiologic correlates of perceived therapist empathy and social-emotional process during psychotherapy. *The Journal of Nervous and Mental Disease, 195*(2), 103–111. https://psycnet.apa.org/doi/10.1097/01.nmd.0000253731.71025.fc

Markon, K. E., Chmielewski, M., & Miller, C. J. (2011). The reliability and validity of discrete and continuous measures of psychopathology: A quantitative review. *Psychological Bulletin, 137*(5), 856–879. https://doi.org/10.1037/a0023678

Mattick, R. P., & Clarke, J. C. (1998). Development and validation of measures of social phobia scrutiny fear and social interaction anxiety. *Behaviour Research and Therapy, 36*(4), 455–470. https://doi.org/10.1016/S0005-7967(97)10031-6

McCarty, C. A., & Weisz, J. R. (2002). Correlates of expressed emotion in mothers of clinically-referred youth: An examination of the five-minute speech sample. *Journal of Child Psychology and Psychiatry, 43*(6), 759–768. https://doi.org/10.1111/1469-7610.00090

McLeod, B. D., Porter, N., Hogue, A., Becker-Haimes, E., & Jensen-Doss, A. (2023). What is the status of multi-informant treatment fidelity research? *Journal of Clinical Child and Adolescent Psychology, 52*(1), 74–94. https://doi.org/10.1080/15374416.2022.2151713

Mian, N. D., Carter, A. S., Pine, D. S., Wakschlag, L. S., & Briggs-Gowan, M. J. (2015). Development of a novel observational measure for anxiety in young children: The Anxiety Dimensional Observation Scale. *Journal of Child Psychology and Psychiatry, 56*(9), 1017–1025. https://doi.org/10.1111/jcpp.12407

Okuno, H., Rezeppa, T., Raskin, T., & De Los Reyes, A. (2022). Adolescent safety behaviors and social anxiety: Links to psychosocial impairments and functioning with unfamiliar peer confederates. *Behavior Modification, 46*(6), 1314–1345. https://doi.org/10.1177/01454455211054019

Pascual, A., Moyano Muñoz, N., & Quílez Robres, A. (2019). The relationship between executive functions and academic performance in primary education: Review and meta-analysis. *Frontiers in Psychology, 10*, 1582. https://doi.org/10.3389/fpsyg.2019.01582

Peters, L., Sunderland, M., Andrews, G., Rapee, R. M., & Mattick, R. P. (2012). Development of a short form Social Interaction Anxiety (SIAS) and Social Phobia Scale (SPS) using nonparametric item response theory: The SIAS-6 and the SPS-6. *Psychological Assessment, 24*(1), 66–76. https://doi.org/10.1037/a0024544

Powers, D. E., & Powers, A. (2015). The incremental contribution of TOEIC® listening, reading, speaking, and writing tests to predicting performance on real-life English language tasks. *Language Testing, 32*(2), 151–167. https://doi.org/10.1177/0265532214551855

Qasmieh, N., Makol, B. A., Augenstein, T. M., Lipton, M. F., Deros, D. E., Karp, J., Keeley, L. M., Truong, M., Racz, S. J., & De Los Reyes, A. (2018). A multi-informant approach to assessing safety behaviors among adolescents: Psychometric properties of the Subtle Avoidance Frequency Examination. *Journal of Child and Family Studies, 27*(6), 1830–1843. https://doi.org/10.1007/s10826-018-1040-5

Racz, S. J., Qasmieh, N., & De Los Reyes, A. (2024). Bivalent fears of evaluation: A developmentally-informed, multi-informant, and multi-modal examination of associations with safety behaviors. *Journal of Anxiety Disorders, 103*, 102846. https://doi.org/10.1016/j.janxdis.2024.102846

Rausch, E., Racz, S. J., Augenstein, T. M., Keeley, L., Lipton, M. F., Szollos, S., Riffle, J., Moriarity, D., Kromash, R., & De Los Reyes, A. (2017). A multi-informant approach to measuring depressive symptoms in clinical assessments of adolescent social anxiety using the Beck Depression Inventory-II: Convergent, incremental, and criterion-related validity. *Child and Youth Care Forum, 46*(5), 661–683. https://doi.org/10.1007/s10566-017-9403-4

Rescorla, R. A., & Wagner, A. R. (1972). A theory of Pavlovian conditioning: variations in the effectiveness of reinforcement and non-reinforcement. In A. H. Prokasy (Ed.), *Classical conditioning II: Current research and theory* (pp. 64–99). Appleton-Century-Croft.

Rezeppa, T., Okuno, H., Qasmieh, N., Racz, S. J., Borelli, J. L., & De Los Reyes, A. (2021). Unfamiliar untrained observers' ratings of adolescent safety behaviors within social interactions with unfamiliar peer confederates. *Behavior Therapy, 52*(3), 564–576. https://doi.org/10.1016/j.beth.2020.07.006

Sangraula, A., & De Los Reyes, A. (2024). Quality of life of parents seeking mental health services for their adolescent's social anxiety: Psychometric properties of the Quality of Life Enjoyment and Satisfaction Questionnaire-Short Form. *Child and Youth Care Forum, 53*(3), 611–629. https://doi.org/10.1007/s10566-023-09770-9

Sewart, A. R., & Craske, M. G. (2020). Inhibitory learning. In J. S. Abramowitz & S. M. Blakey (Eds.), *Clinical handbook of fear and anxiety: Maintenance processes and treatment mechanisms* (pp. 265–285). American Psychological Association.

Sher-Censor, E. (2015). Five Minute Speech Sample in developmental research: A review. *Developmental Review, 36*, 127–155. https://doi.org/10.1016/j.dr.2015.01.005

Silk, J. S., Stroud, L. R., Siegle, G. J., Dahl, R. E., Lee, K. H., & Nelson, E. E. (2012). Peer acceptance and rejection through the eyes of youth: Pupillary, eyetracking and ecological data from the Chatroom Interact Task. *Social Cognitive and Affective Neuroscience, 7*(1), 93–105. https://doi.org/10.1093/scan/nsr044

Skinner, B. F. (1953). *Science and human behavior*. Macmillan.

Smith, G. T., Fischer, S., & Fister, S. M. (2003). Incremental validity principles in test construction. *Psychological Assessment, 15*(4), 467–477. https://doi.org/10.1037/1040-3590.15.4.467

Steinglass, P. (1979). The Home Observation Assessment Method (HOAM): Real-time naturalistic observation of families in their homes. *Family Process, 18*(3), 337–354. https://doi.org/10.1111/j.1545-5300.1979.00337.x

Szollos, S., Keeley, L. M., Makol, B. A., Weeks, J. W., Racz, S. J., Lipton, M. F., Augenstein, T. M., Beale, A. M., & De Los Reyes, A. (2019). Multi-informant assessments of individual differences in adolescents' socio-evaluative fears: Clinical correlates and links to arousal within social interactions. *Journal of Child and Family Studies, 28*(12), 3360–3373. https://doi.org/10.1007/s10826-019-01517-2

Talbott, E., De Los Reyes, A., Kearns, D. M., Mancilla-Martinez, J., Cook, C. R., & Wang, M. (2023). Evidence-based assessment in special education research: Advancing the use of evidence in assessment tools and empirical processes. *Exceptional Children, 89*(4), 467–487. https://doi.org/10.1177/00144029231171092

Tesh, E. M., & Holditch-Davis, D. (1997). HOME inventory and NCATS: Relation to mother and child behaviors during naturalistic observations. *Research in Nursing & Health, 20*(4), 295–307. https://doi.org/10.1002/(SICI)1098-240X(199708)20:4%3C295::AID-NUR3%3E3.0.CO;2-B

Thomas, S. A., Jain, A., Wilson, T., Deros, D. E., Jacobs, I., Dunn, E. J., Aldao, A., Stadnik, R., & De Los Reyes, A. (2019). Moderated mediation of the link between parent-adolescent conflict and adolescent risk-taking: The role of physiological regulation and hostile behavior in an experimentally controlled investigation. *Journal of Psychopathology and Behavioral Assessment, 41*(4), 699–715. https://doi.org/10.1007/s10862-019-09747-w

Vlachou, M., Andreou, E., & Botsoglou, K. (2014). Bully/victim problems among preschool children: Naturalistic observations in the classroom and on the playground. *International Journal of Learning: Annual Review, 20*(1), 77–93. https://doi.org/10.18848/1447-9494/CGP/v20/48734

Wakschlag, L. S., Briggs-Gowan, M. J., Hill, C., Danis, B., Leventhal, B. L., Keenan, K., Egger, H. L., Cicchetti, D., Burns, J., & Carter, A. S. (2008). Observational assessment of preschool disruptive behavior, Part 2: Validity of the Disruptive Behavior Diagnostic Observation Schedule (DB-DOS). *Journal of the American Academy of Child and Adolescent Psychiatry, 47*(6), 632–641. https://doi.org/10.1097/CHI.0b013e31816c5c10

Wakschlag, L. S., Tolan, P. H., & Leventhal, B. L. (2010). Research review: "Ain't misbehavin:" Towards a developmentally-specified nosology for preschool disruptive behavior. *Journal of Child Psychology and Psychiatry, 51*(1), 3–22. https://doi.org/10.1111/j.1469-7610.2009.02184.x

Wang, Y. P., & Gorenstein, C. (2013). Psychometric properties of the Beck Depression Inventory-II: A comprehensive review. *Revista Brasileira de Psiquiatria, 35*(4), 416–431. https://doi.org/10.1590/1516-4446-2012-1048

Watts, A. L., Makol, B. A., Palumbo, I. M., De Los Reyes, A., Olino, T. M., Latzman, R. D., DeYoung, C. G., Wood, P. K., & Sher, K. J. (2022). How robust is the p-factor? Using multitrait-multimethod modeling to inform the meaning of general factors of psychopathology in youth. *Clinical Psychological Science, 10*(4), 640–661. https://doi.org/10.1177/21677026211055170

Weisz, J. R., & Kazdin, A. E. (2017). The present and future of evidence-based psychotherapies for children and adolescents. In J. R. Weisz & A. E. Kazdin (Eds.), *Evidence-based psychotherapies for children and adolescents* (3rd ed., pp. 577–595). Guilford.

Zhang, S., & Zhang, X. (2022). The relationship between vocabulary knowledge and L2 reading/listening comprehension: A meta-analysis. *Language Teaching Research, 26*(4), 696–725. https://doi.org/10.1177/1362168820913998

Chapter 7
Criterion-Related Validation Test of Strategies for Integrating Behavioral Data in Youth Development

As we argued in Chap. 6, findings from criterion-related validation studies complement the findings from Monte Carlo simulations of validity performance that we reported in Chap. 5. Criterion-related validation studies provide us with a naturalistic test of the performance of integrative strategies like the Satellite Model and the Trifactor Model. Specifically, we require tests of these models when applied to multi-informant data that vary in their relations to validity criteria. Consider the assumptions of both the Satellite Model and the Trifactor Model. The former model assumes that common variance and unique variance may each contain valid data. The latter model assumes that only common variance contains valid data. In essence, these models vary in sources of valid data—two sources versus one source. Thus, how do these integrative strategies perform when applied to a real-world scenario in which (a) multiple informants' reports produce discrepant results; (b) among these informants, a single informant (i.e., unique variance) outperforms the others when predicting a validity criterion; and (c) the variance informants share (i.e., common variance) has predictive value as well?

The criterion-related validation study we described in Chap. 6 is ideally suited to address this larger question. The study focused on a behavioral domain that, among adolescents, tends to display considerable variation within and across social contexts (i.e., social anxiety; see Alfano & Beidel, 2011). Further, the validity criteria used in the study (i.e., simulated social interactions among adolescents and same-age, unfamiliar peers) were designed to reference behaviors that manifest in a single, domain-relevant context, namely, peer interactions that occur outside of the home (Cannon et al., 2020). Prior work supports this design feature of the study. Adolescents' behavior within these interactions references contexts that caregivers are relatively unlikely to observe in day-to-day life (see Charamut et al., 2022; Deros et al., 2018; Keeley et al., 2024). Taken together, the design of the validity criteria, coupled with the informants involved in the assessment (i.e., caregivers, adolescents, peer confederates), creates a scenario in which informants vary in their ability to predict criterion variables. In fact, within Project CONTEXT, peer

B. A. Makol et al., *Youth Development in Context*, Springer Series on Child and Family Studies, https://doi.org/10.1007/978-3-031-80549-3_7

confederate reports outperform caregiver and adolescent reports when predicting observed anxiety within peer interactions (see Glenn et al., 2019). As noted in Chap. 6, studies like Project CONTEXT exemplify a common practice among scholars in youth development—the use of context-sensitive instruments to represent behavioral domains (Table 6.2). As such, it also provides a conservative test of the modeling assumptions of both the Satellite Model and the Trifactor Model. This chapter describes the analytic plan we used to address our Study 2 aims and reports the findings of this study.

7.1 Study 2 Aims and Data Analytic Plan

7.1.1 Preliminary Analyses

We conducted analyses to determine whether the data used in Study 2 met the basic assumptions of parametric statistical tests (i.e., skewness/kurtosis in the range of ±2.0). In addition, we computed bivariate correlations to examine relations within and between informants' reports of adolescent social anxiety.

7.1.2 Aim 1: Implementing the Trifactor Model

We implemented four Trifactor Models using Mplus Version 8.5, including models for caregiver-adolescent reports, caregiver-peer reports, adolescent-peer reports, and caregiver-adolescent-peer reports on the SPS-6 (see Figs. 7.1 and 7.2). For each Trifactor Model, we strictly followed the model-building procedures described by Bauer et al. (2013) and used full-information maximum likelihood estimation to calculate likelihood ratio tests and score estimates. We identified each factor through imposing a set of constraints on the factor loadings and factor correlations. First, all informants' ratings were loaded onto the *Common Factor*. The *Common Factor* reflects informants' shared variability in item ratings of adolescent social anxiety. Second, we loaded each informant's reports onto the appropriate *Perspective Factor* (i.e., one per informant). The informants included in this study consistently provide reports that correlate at low-to-moderate magnitudes (Achenbach et al., 1987; De Los Reyes et al., 2015). Further, prior work supports the notion that these informants vary according to their unique contexts and perspectives when rating youth anxiety (Cannon et al., 2020; Deros et al., 2018; Etkin et al., 2021a, b). Thus, we modeled these informants as structurally different. Consistent with Bauer et al.'s (2013) recommendations for structurally different informants, we equated the intercept and factor loading across informants for the first SPS-6 item (i.e., Item 4) and freely estimated the intercepts and factor loadings for the remaining items. Third, we regressed *Specific Factors* onto parallel SPS-6 items completed by informants.

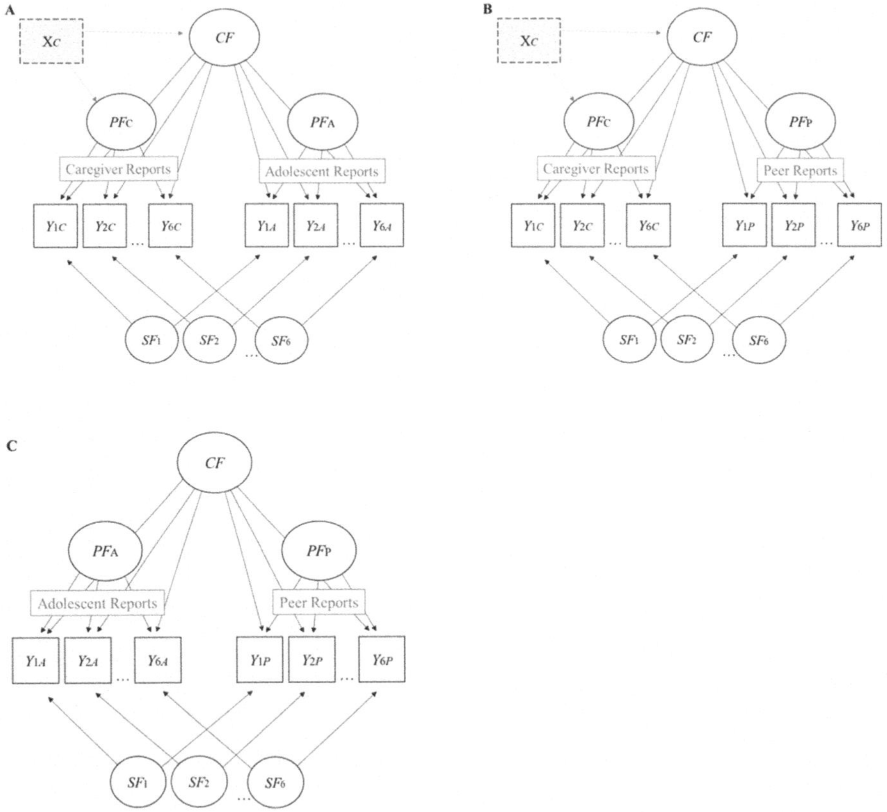

Fig. 7.1 Unconditional and Conditional Trifactor Models (Trifactor Models) using multi-informant reports of adolescent social anxiety on the six-item short form of the Social Phobia Scale (SPS-6). Panel A represents the caregiver-adolescent report model, Panel B represents the caregiver-peer report model, and Panel C represents the adolescent-peer report model. Observed item ratings are numbered by item. *C*, *A*, and *P* subscripts are for caregiver, adolescent, and peer confederate ratings, respectively. The *Common Factor* (CF), *Perspective Factors* (*PFs*), and *Specific Factors* (*SFs*) are modeled from observed item ratings. Dashed lines indicate additional model inputs in the Conditional Trifactor Models (Panel A and Panel B). The informant-specific predictor, caregiver self-reported depressive symptoms, is denoted with an X_C and is loaded onto the caregiver PF as well as the CF. (Figures adapted from Bauer et al., 2013)

We modeled all latent factors (i.e., *Common*, *Perspective*, *Specific Factors*) as orthogonal to each other. Models that included caregiver reports of adolescent social anxiety represented Conditional Trifactor Models given that they included an informant-level predictor (caregiver self-reports of depressive symptoms) consistent with the depression→distortion hypothesis (Richters, 1992) and Bauer et al.'s (2013) original application of the Trifactor Model. Specifically, we regressed caregiver BDI-II reports onto the *Common* Factor and caregiver *Perspective Factor*.

Consistent with Bauer et al.'s (2013) recommendations, we placed additional constraints on the models to set the scale of the latent variables. For the Unconditional

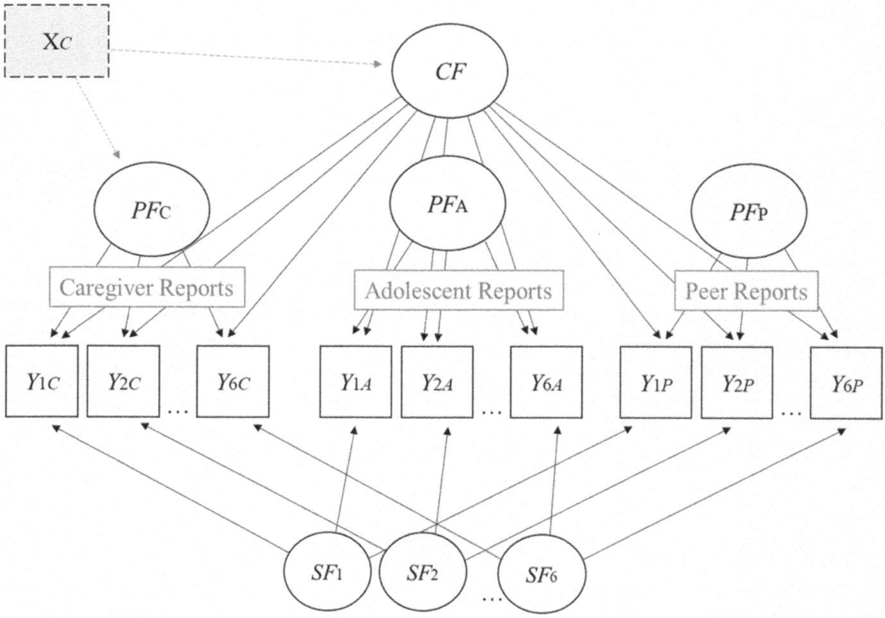

Fig. 7.2 Conditional Trifactor Model (Trifactor Model) using caregiver, adolescent, and peer confederate reports of adolescent social anxiety on the six-item short form of the Social Phobia Scale (SPS-6). Observed item ratings are numbered by item. *C*, *A*, and *P* subscripts are for caregiver, adolescent, and peer confederate ratings, respectively. The *Common Factor* (CF), *Perspective Factors* (*PFs*), and Specific Factors (*SFs*) are modeled from observed item ratings. The informant-specific predictor, caregiver self-reported depressive symptoms, is denoted with an X_C and is loaded onto the caregiver PF as well as the CF. (Figures adapted from Bauer et al., 2013)

Trifactor Model, we set the means and variances of the *Common*, *Perspective*, and *Specific Factors* to 0 and 1, respectively. Doing so allowed for all nonzero factor loadings to be estimated and interpreted in terms of their relative magnitude. For the Conditional Trifactor Models, we set the intercepts and residual variances of the *Common Factor*, *Perspective Factors*, and *Specific Factors* to 0 and 1, respectively.

For the final converged models, we evaluated model fit indices. These indices included the Steiger-Lind Root-Mean-Square Error of Approximation (RMSEA; Steiger, 1990), Bentler Comparative Fit Index (CFI; Bentler, 1990), and Tucker-Lewis Index (TLI; Tucker & Lewis, 1973). We considered model fit acceptable if the following model fit criteria were met: RMSEA $\leq$0.06, CFI $\geq$ 0.95, and TLI $\geq$ 0.95 (Hu & Bentler, 1999; Kline, 2016; McDonald & Ho, 2002). For converged Trifactor Models with satisfactory model fit, we calculated integrated multi-informant factor scores for use in subsequent analyses. Consistent with Curran et al. (2020), factor scores for the *Common*, *Perspective*, and *Specific Factors* were estimated as maximum likelihood expected a posteriori (EAP) scores. This approach up-weights items that are more strongly related to the factor and down-weights those that are less strongly related to the factor.

7.1.3 Aim 2: Implementing the Satellite Model

We implemented the Satellite Model in SPSS Version 24 by applying principal components analysis to caregiver, adolescent, and peer confederate SIAS reports. Consistent with Kraemer et al. (2003), we conducted an unrotated principal components analysis with the number of components extracted set to three. We evaluated component weights to determine whether the first component was consistent with a *Trait* score (i.e., component weights loading strongly and in the same direction). We used factor analytic criteria to decide whether to retain the three-component principal components analysis: Bartlett's Test of Sphericity is significant (Bartlett, 1950), Kaiser-Meyer-Olkin test (KMO) $\geq .60$ (Kaiser, 1970), and the first component (i.e., *Trait* score) eigenvalue > 1 (Pett et al., 2003).

7.1.4 Aim 3: Incremental Validity Relative to Individual Informants' Reports and the Composite Score

We tested the incremental validity of the Trifactor Model *Common Factor* using a series of hierarchical linear and logistic regressions. Consistent with well-established incremental validity conventions (Garb, 2003; Hunsley & Meyer, 2003; Smith et al., 2003), we benchmarked the ability of *Common Factor* scores to explain variance in criterion variables, relative to well-established strategies for analyzing multi-informant data (i.e., individually, composite score). In separate regressions, we evaluated whether the *Common Factor* scores explained variance in adolescent referral status and observed adolescent social anxiety, over and above the explanatory value of individual informants' reports or the composite score (i.e., models involved either individual informants' reports or the composite score, but not both simultaneously). In separate regression models, we added caregiver (i.e., SPAIC), adolescent (i.e., SPAIC), and peer confederate (i.e., SIAS) reports of adolescent social anxiety in the first step as independent variables. Using a similar design, we ran separate regression models in which the composite score (using averages from informants' SIAS reports) was added in the first step as an independent variable. We only ran these regression models for scores from Trifactor Models that included the informants' reports both individually and when averaged. For instance, we included caregiver SPAIC reports in regression models evaluating the incremental validity of the caregiver-adolescent *Common Factor* score, but not in the regression model evaluating the incremental validity of the adolescent-peer *Common Factor* score. We included observed adolescent social anxiety and adolescent referral status (0 = community control, 1 = clinic-referred) as dependent variables in these models. We ran separate models for each *Common Factor* score, alternative integrative strategy, and dependent variable.

Similarly, we tested the incremental validity of the Satellite Model *Trait* score relative to individual informants' reports and the composite score using a series of hierarchical linear and logistic regressions. These regressions evaluated whether the *Trait* score explained variance in adolescent referral status and observed adolescent social anxiety, over and above the explanatory value of individual informants' reports and the composite score. In separate regression models, we added caregiver (i.e., SPAIC), adolescent (i.e., SPAIC), and peer confederate (i.e., SPS) reports of adolescent social anxiety in the first step as independent variables. Using a similar design, we ran separate regression models for each composite score (using averages from informants' SPS reports) in the first step as independent variables. We included observed adolescent social anxiety and adolescent referral status (0 = community control, 1 = clinic-referred) as dependent variables in these models. We ran separate models for each alternative integrative strategy and dependent variable. Of note, we previously conducted a subset of these analyses using a smaller version of the same sample, namely, tests of the Satellite Model (i.e., Makol et al., 2020). For the current study, we re-ran the analyses focused on the Satellite Model to allow for a direct comparison of the effects obtained in criterion-related and incremental validity analyses examining the Trifactor Model *Common Factor* and Satellite Model *Trait* scores.

7.1.5 Aim 4: Directly Comparing the Incremental Validity of Scores Derived from the Trifactor Model and Satellite Model

We evaluated the incremental validity of the Trifactor Model *Common Factor* score using caregiver, adolescent, and peer confederate reports relative to the Satellite Model *Trait* score using two hierarchical linear and logistic regressions. These regressions evaluated whether the *Common Factor* score explained variance in adolescent referral status and observed adolescent social anxiety, over and above the explanatory value of the *Trait* score. We entered the *Trait* score in the first step as an independent variable and the *Common Factor* score in the second step as an independent variable. We then conducted an additional set of regression models in which the *Common Factor* score was added in the first step as an independent variable, and the *Trait* score was added in the second step as an independent variable. We only compared these two scores, because it allowed for a comparison of scores derived from the Trifactor Model and Satellite Model when both models leveraged the same three informants. Dependent variables included observed adolescent social anxiety and adolescent referral status (0 = community control, 1 = clinic-referred). We ran a separate model for each order of entering the independent variables and dependent variables.

For all aims, we interpreted statistical significance for analyses using a p-value threshold of <0.05. We inferred magnitudes of effect sizes based on Cohen's (1988) effect size conventions for the effect size r and β (low: 0.10; moderate: 0.30; large: 0.50). Unlike the exploratory demographic comparison analyses reported in Chap.

6, we did not apply Bonferroni's corrections to the analyses reported below. This decision is consistent with recommendations on the judicious use of Bonferroni's corrections (Armstrong, 2014; Streiner & Norman, 2011).

7.2 Study 2 Results and Discussion

7.2.1 Preliminary Analyses

Descriptive statistics for all Study 2 measures are included in Table 7.1. As mentioned previously, all informants' survey reports displayed acceptable levels of internal consistency, and all independent observers' ratings displayed acceptable levels of inter-rater reliability. Further, with the exception of caregiver self-reports of depression on the BDI-II, all measures displayed acceptable levels of skewness and kurtosis. We applied a square root transformation to caregiver BDI-II reports, which reduced kurtosis to tolerable levels. The transformed BDI-II reports were used in the analyses described below.

Table 7.1 Descriptive statistics for caregiver, adolescent, and peer confederate survey measures (Study 2)

Variable	*N*	Mean	Standard deviation	Skewness	Kurtosis
SPS-6					
Adolescent self-report	134	6.19	5.59	1.25	0.91
Caregiver report	134	4.77	5.14	1.21	0.45
Peer confederate report	131	8.48	5.68	0.41	−0.59
SIAS					
Adolescent self-report	134	28.05	16.14	0.84	0.17
Caregiver report	134	27.04	16.54	0.77	0.02
Peer confederate report	132	35.55	17.51	0.09	−0.99
SPAI-C					
Adolescent self-report	134	17.39	10.58	0.62	−0.23
Caregiver report	134	17.45	10.91	0.61	−0.28
SPS					
Adolescent self-report	134	21.42	15.41	1.28	1.47
Caregiver report	134	16.91	14.39	1.18	0.72
Peer confederate report	131	25.83	16.63	0.59	−0.25
BDI-II					
Caregiver self-report, raw score	134	8.69	8.31	1.49	3.04
Caregiver self-report, square root transformation	134	2.54	1.50	0.08	−0.38

Note: *SPS-6* Social Phobia Scale 6-item Short Form, *SIAS* Social Interaction Anxiety Scale, *SPAIC* Social Phobia and Anxiety Inventory for Children, *SIAS* Social Interaction Anxiety Scale, *SPS* Social Phobia Scale, *BDI-II* Beck Depression Inventory-II

Table 7.2 Correlations among caregiver, adolescent, and peer confederate reports used for integrative strategies tested (Study 2)

Measure, informant	1	2	3	4	5	6
1. **SPS-6**, adolescent self-report	–	0.31***	0.38***	0.80***	0.34***	0.48***
2. **SPS-6**, caregiver		–	0.01	0.31***	0.73***	0.13
3. **SPS-6**, peer confederate			–	0.29**	0.18*	0.82***
4. **SIAS**, adolescent self-report				–	0.39***	0.42***
5. **SIAS**, caregiver					–	0.30***
6. **SIAS**, peer confederate						–

Note: Boxes denote correlations between informants on parallel surveys used in Study 2 integrative strategies. *SPS-6* Social Phobia Scale 6-item Short Form, *SIAS* Social Interaction Anxiety Scale; *$p < .05$; **$p < .01$; ***$p < .001$

In Table 7.2, we reported bivariate correlations among informants' reports on social anxiety measures used in the Satellite Model and the Trifactor Model. Overall, correlations between informants' reports on the same social anxiety measure were in the moderate-magnitude range, consistent with levels of correspondence in the larger cross-informant literature (Achenbach et al., 1987; De Los Reyes et al., 2015). However, consistent with prior research (Deros et al., 2018), the correlation between caregiver and peer confederate reports on the SPS-6 was near-zero in magnitude and non-significant.

7.2.2 *Aim 1: Implementing the Trifactor Model*

We implemented the Trifactor Models using model-building procedures described by Bauer et al. (2013) and as detailed previously. Across Trifactor Models, we entered SPS-6 reports into the model for each informant. For Conditional Trifactor Models, we regressed the informant-specific predictor (caregiver self-reported depressive symptoms on the BDI-II) onto the *Common Factor* and caregiver *Perspective Factor*. When describing model findings, we interpreted the standardized factor loadings given that they are directly comparable when understanding the relative effects of the *Common*, *Perspective*, and *Specific Factors* on informants' SPS-6 items.

7.2.2.1 Adolescent-Peer Trifactor Model

We implemented the Unconditional Trifactor Model using adolescent and peer confederate SPS-6 reports as shown in Fig. 7.1 (Panel C). The initial model converged, and fit criteria indicated mixed but overall acceptable fit of the model to the data, $\chi^2(38) = 60.79$, $p < 0.05$; RMSEA = 0.07, 90% CI [0.03, 0.10]; CFI = 0.97; TLI = 0.95. We retained this model and reported raw and standardized intercept and factor loading estimates in Tables 7.3 and 7.4. Both adolescent and peer confederate

Table 7.3 Raw intercept and factor loading estimates for the unconditional adolescent-peer confederate Trifactor Model implemented in Study 2

Raw estimates							
	Intercept		Common factor		Perspective factor		
Item	P	A	P	A	P	A	Specific factor[a]
4	1.65***		0.46***	0.90***	0.86***		−0.26
7	1.17***	1.02***	0.22*	0.82***	0.65***	0.26	−0.35**
8	1.50***	1.06***	0.40***	1.05***	0.97***	−0.01	0.27**
15	1.22***	1.00***	0.30**	0.74***	0.72***	0.10	0.39***
16	1.58***	0.92***	0.27*	0.94***	0.89***	−0.12	0.20
17	1.06***	0.66***	0.42***	0.63***	0.83***	−0.16	0.17

Note. [a]All *Specific Factor* loadings are within 0.03 between informants. When different, the peer confederate's loadings are reported. *P* Peer, *A* Adolescent; *$p < 0.05$; **$p < 0.01$; ***$p < 0.001$

Table 7.4 Standardized intercept and factor loading estimates for the unconditional adolescent-peer confederate Trifactor Model implemented in Study 2

Standardized estimates							
	Intercept		Common factor		Perspective factor		
Item	P	A	P	A	P	A	Specific factor[a]
4	1.30***		0.37***	0.69***	0.68***	0.67***	−0.21
7	1.00***	0.79***	0.19*	0.63***	0.56***	0.20	−0.30**
8	1.25***	0.85***	0.33***	0.84***	81***	−0.01	−0.23**
15	1.12***	0.91***	0.27**	0.67***	0.66***	0.09	0.35***
16	1.37***	0.80***	0.23**	0.82***	0.77***	−0.10	0.17
17	0.99***	0.72***	0.39***	0.68***	0.77***	−0.18	0.16

Note. [a]All *Specific Factor* loadings are within 0.03 between informants. When different, the peer confederate's loadings are reported. *P* Peer, *A* Adolescent; *$p < 0.05$; **$p < 0.01$; ***$p < 0.001$

reports loaded significantly and positively onto the *Common Factor*, with adolescent self-reports exhibiting stronger loadings (0.63–0.84 vs. 0.19–0.39). Peer confederate reports loaded positively and strongly onto the peer *Perspective Factor* (0.56–0.81). In contrast, adolescent self-reports did not load significantly onto the adolescent *Perspective Factor* with the exception of Item 4 ("Nervous people are staring"). We observed significant and negative loadings onto *Specific Factors* for Item 7 ("Worries about shaking or trembling") and Item 8 ("Gets tense when facing others"), as well as a significant and positive loading for the *Specific Factor* for Item 15 ("Worries about attracting attention").

7.2.2.2 Caregiver-Adolescent Trifactor Model

We implemented the Conditional Trifactor Model using caregiver and adolescent SPS-6 reports as shown in Fig. 7.1 (Panel A). The initial model converged, and fit criteria suggested a good model fit to the data, $\chi^2(46) = 42.72$, $p = 0.61$; RMSEA = 0.00, 90% CI [0.00, 0.05]; CFI = 1.00; TLI = 1.00. We retained this

Table 7.5 Raw intercept and factor loading estimates for the conditional caregiver-adolescent Trifactor Model implemented in Study 2

Raw estimates							
	Intercept		Common factor		Perspective factor		
Item	C	A	C	A	C	A	Specific factor[a]
4	4.24		0.30**	0.82**	0.76***		−0.10
7	3.39	4.65	0.16	0.74**	0.46***	0.81**	0.25*
8	4.27	4.40	0.33**	0.99***	0.81***	0.24	−0.09
15	3.09	2.55	0.26**	0.72***	0.73****	0.41	−0.30***
16	5.53	5.53	0.33**	1.08***	0.90***	−0.20	0.18
17	3.36	2.21	0.35***	0.64***	0.71***	0.13	−0.22*

Note. [a]When *Specific Factor* loadings are within 0.03 between informants, the caregiver's loadings are reported. When greater than 0.03, the loadings for each informant are reported. *C* Caregiver, *A* Adolescent; **p* < 0.05; ***p* < 0.01; ****p* < 0.001

Table 7.6 Standardized intercept and factor loading estimates for the conditional caregiver-adolescent Trifactor Model (Study 2)

Standardized estimates								
	Intercept		Common factor		Perspective factor		Specific factor[a]	
Item	C	A	C	A	C	A	C	A
4	3.56	3.22	0.26**	0.62***	0.66***	0.45	−0.09	
7	3.93	3.59	0.18	0.57**	0.55***	0.49	0.29*	0.19*
8	3.94	3.52	0.31***	0.80****	0.78***	0.15	−0.08	
15	2.96	2.30	0.25**	0.65***	0.73***	0.29	−0.29***	
16	4.86	4.79	0.29**	0.93***	0.83***	−0.14	0.15	
17	3.32	2.31	0.34***	0.66***	0.73***	0.11	−0.22*	

Note: [a]When *Specific Factor* loadings are within 0.03 between informants, the caregiver's loadings are reported. When greater than 0.03, the loadings for each informant are reported. *C* Caregiver, *A* Adolescent; **p* < 0.05; ***p* < 0.01; ****p* < 0.001

model and reported raw and standardized intercept and factor loading estimates in Tables 7.5 and 7.6. Adolescent self-reports loaded positively and significantly onto the *Common Factor* (0.57–0.93). Caregiver reports loaded positively but less strongly onto the *Common Factor* (0.18–0.34), with the exception of Item 7 ("Worries about shaking or trembling", $p = 0.051$). Whereas caregiver reports loaded significantly and positively onto the caregiver *Perspective Factor* (0.55–0.83), adolescent self-reports did not load significantly onto the adolescent *Perspective Factor* (−0.14–0.49). We observed significant and negative *Specific Factor* loadings for Item 7 ("Worries about shaking or trembling"), Item 15 ("Worries about attracting attention"), and Item 17 ("Feels conspicuous standing in line"). The informant-specific predictor (caregiver self-reported depressive symptoms) was significantly related to the caregiver *Perspective Factor* ($\beta = 0.28$, standard error [SE] = 0.09, $p < 0.01$) but did not relate to the *Common Factor* ($\beta = -0.03$, SE = 0.09, $p = 0.75$). This suggests that as caregivers' self-reported depressive symptoms increased, they were more likely to rate their adolescent's social anxiety higher, which is captured by the predictor's specific impact on the unique variance in the caregivers' social anxiety reports that is explained by their *Perspective Factor*. One might interpret this effect as reflecting "rater bias" consistent with the depression→distortion hypothesis. The validation tests reported below probe this interpretation. That is, if this model partials out variance reflected by rater bias, then presumably the model should perform quite well not just when compared to the individual informant's report (i.e., caregiver), but also to the Satellite Model, which does not treat this unique variance as rater bias.

7.2.2.3 Caregiver-Peer Trifactor Model

We implemented the Conditional Trifactor Model using caregiver and peer confederate SPS-6 reports as shown in Fig. 7.1 (Panel B). The initial model did not converge due to a non-positive definite covariance matrix. We modified model constraints for problematic parameters (including setting the residual variance of the peer confederates' Item 4 and Item 7 reports and caregivers' Item 7 reports to a near-zero, positive value), which allowed the model to converge but resulted in poor model fit, $\chi^2(49) = 122.66$, $p < 0.001$; RMSEA = 0.11, 90% CI [0.08, 0.13]; CFI = 0.92; TLI = 0.86. We thus modified various model constraints to improve model fit, which was unsuccessful. Given these model fit issues, we did not retain the caregiver-peer Trifactor Model or use it in subsequent analyses examining the validity of the *Common Factor* scores.

7.2.2.4 Caregiver-Adolescent-Peer Trifactor Model

We implemented the Conditional Trifactor Model using caregiver, adolescent, and peer confederate SPS-6 reports as shown in Fig. 7.2. The initial model did not converge due to a non-positive definite covariance matrix. Given that the variance in peer confederates' Item 4 reports was almost completely explained by the latent factors in the model, we set the residual variance for this item to a near-zero, positive value. This resulted in a positive-definite and converged model with overall good model fit, with the exception of the chi-square test of model fit, $\chi^2(129) = 169.39$, $p < 0.01$; RMSEA = 0.05, 90% CI [0.03, 0.07]; CFI = 0.97; TLI = 0.96. We retained this model and reported raw and standardized intercept and factor loading estimates in Tables 7.7 and 7.8. Adolescent and peer confederate reports loaded positively and significantly onto the *Common Factor* (0.29–0.77), with the exception of adolescent self-reports on Item 17 ("Feels conspicuous standing in line"). In contrast, caregiver reports did not load significantly onto the *Common Factor* (−0.02–0.08), although they loaded positively and significantly onto the caregiver *Perspective Factor* (0.58–0.87). Thus, a notable feature of this application of the Trifactor Model is that the *Common Factor* primarily weights adolescent and peer confederate reports, with a non-significant contribution from caregiver reports, which are instead captured primarily in the caregiver *Perspective Factor*. Both adolescent and peer

Table 7.7 Raw intercept and factor loading estimates for the conditional three-informant Trifactor Model implemented in Study 2

Raw estimates

	Intercept			Common factor			Perspective factor			Specific factor[a]
Item	C	P	A	C	P	A	C	P	A	
4	2.92**			0.10	0.40*	0.43*	0.81***			0.23*
7	1.37	2.42**	1.96*	−0.02	0.51***	0.37*	0.49***	0.29**	0.77***	0.11
8	1.78*	2.80**	1.50**	0.03	0.82***	0.41*	0.87***	0.38***	0.97***	−0.20**
15	2.60*	3.22*	2.47*	0.01	0.71***	0.46***	0.78***	0.25**	0.65***	0.29***
16	1.85*	2.88**	1.21**	0.01	0.84***	0.35**	0.96***	0.23*	0.88***	−0.22**
17	2.43*	3.15*	1.48*	0.06	0.80***	0.18	0.81***	0.29**	0.57***	0.24***

Note. [a]All *Specific Factor* loadings are within 0.04. When different, the peer confederate's loadings are reported. *C* Caregiver, *P* Peer, *A* Adolescent; $p < 0.05$; $^{**}p < 0.01$; $^{***}p < 0.001$

Table 7.8 Standardized intercept and factor loading estimates for the conditional three-informant Trifactor Model (Study 2)

Standardized estimates

	Intercept			Common factor			Perspective factor			Specific factor[a]
Item	C	P	A	C	P	A	C	P	A	
4	2.43**	2.36**	2.21**	0.08	0.32*	0.32**	0.70***	0.93***	0.62***	0.18*
7	1.58	2.10**	1.51*	−0.02	0.44***	0.29*	0.58***	0.36**	0.60***	0.09
8	1.63*	2.41**	1.18**	0.03	0.71***	0.32**	0.83***	0.47**	0.78***	−0.17**
15	2.49*	2.95*	2.21**	0.01	0.65***	0.41***	0.77***	0.33*	0.60***	0.26***
16	1.63*	2.56**	1.03**	0.01	0.75***	0.30**	0.87***	0.29	0.76***	−0.19**
17	2.38*	3.03*	1.63*	0.06	0.77***	0.19	0.82***	0.40*	0.64***	0.23***

Note: [a]All *Specific Factor* loadings are within 0.04. When different, the peer confederate's loadings are reported. *C* Caregiver, *P* Peer, *A* Adolescent; $p < 0.05$; $^{**}p < 0.01$; $^{***}p < 0.001$

confederate reports loaded significantly and positively onto their respective *Perspective Factors* (0.33–0.93), with the exception of peer confederates' reports on Item 16 ("Tense in elevator"). A total of five SPS-6 items had significant *Specific Factor* loadings, including positive loadings for Item 4 ("Nervous people are staring"), Item 15 ("Worries about attracting attention"), and Item 17 ("Feels conspicuous standing in line") and negative loadings for Item 8 ("Gets tense facing others") and Item 16 ("Tense in elevator"). Consistent with the caregiver-adolescent model findings, caregiver self-reported depressive symptoms were significantly related to the caregiver *Perspective Factor* ($\beta = 0.26$, SE = 0.09, $p < 0.01$) but did not relate to the *Common Factor* ($\beta = -0.05$, SE = 0.10, $p = 0.61$). This suggests that as caregivers' self-reported depressive symptoms increased, they were more likely to rate their adolescent's social anxiety higher, which is captured by the predictor's specific impact on the unique variance in the caregivers' social anxiety reports that is explained by their *Perspective Factor*. As with the Caregiver-Adolescent Trifactor Model, the interpretation that this relation between caregivers' self-reported depressive symptoms and their adolescent social anxiety reports reflects a rater bias is evaluated using the validation tests reported below.

In sum, model fit and factor loadings for Trifactor Models varied depending on the informants entered into the model and were driven, in part, by the extent to which informants' reports on the SPS-6 displayed a high degree of common variance. For example, caregiver-peer reports were not significantly correlated, and the caregiver-peer Trifactor Model exhibited poor model fit. This supports the notion that the Trifactor Model works particularly well when applied to informants' reports that share, at minimum, a fair degree of common variance. Indeed, adolescent-caregiver and adolescent-peer SPS-6 reports correlated at moderate levels, and Trifactor Models using these dyads resulted in a satisfactory model fit, with both informants' reports loading significantly onto the *Common Factor*. However, in these models, adolescents' reports loaded more strongly onto the *Common Factor* than the adolescent *Perspective Factor*, whereas the reverse was true for caregiver and peer confederate reports. Further, these observations align with findings as to the variable convergence rates of Trifactor Models simulated in Study 2, as well as with issues reported in prior work surrounding sample-specific modifications needed to improve model fit (cf. Bauer et al., 2013; Clark et al., 2017; Makol, 2022; Martel et al., 2017a, b). Collectively, these findings point to a key notion: The Trifactor Model may only yield adequate model fit under data conditions characterized by significant amounts of common variance among reports entered into the model.

7.2.3 Aim 2: Implementing the Satellite Model

Consistent with procedures described by Kraemer et al. (2003), we implemented the Satellite Model using caregiver, adolescent, and peer confederate SIAS reports (see Table 7.9). We entered these reports into an unrotated principal components analysis in which we set the number of components extracted to three. We retained this three-factor solution given that all factor analytic criteria were met including a statistically significant Bartlett's Test of Sphericity ($\chi^2(3) = 50.41$, $p < 0.001$), KMO just above the cutoff of 0.60 (KMO = 0.64), and eigenvalue >1 for the *Trait* score component. Similar to prior work (Kraemer et al., 2003; Makol et al., 2020), we

Table 7.9 Principal components analysis of caregiver, adolescent, and peer confederate reports on the Social Interaction Anxiety Scale (SIAS) (Study 2)

Component:	Trait	Context	Perspective
Informant	Component weight		
Caregiver	0.73	0.63	0.27
Adolescent	0.81	−0.06	−0.59
Peer confederate	0.75	−0.55	0.37
Total variance explained			
Eigenvalue	1.75	0.70	0.56
Variance attributable to component	58.24%	23.25%	18.52%

qualitatively examined the component loadings and found that they were consistent with *Trait* (positive and large in magnitude across informants), *Context* (contrasting loadings for caregiver and peer confederate reports with adolescent reports loading between caregiver and peer confederate reports), and *Perspective* (contrasting loadings for adolescent reports and caregiver and peer confederate reports) scores. Kraemer and colleagues' assumption that this strategy for integrating informants' reports maximizes the variance explained in the reports—and, by extension, optimizes measurement validity—is evaluated through validation testing below.

7.2.4 Aim 3: Incremental Validity Relative to Informants' Reports and the Composite Score

7.2.4.1 Incremental Validity of Scores Derived from the Trifactor Model Relative to Individual Informants' Reports (Tables 7.10 and 7.11)

We conducted hierarchical regression analyses to determine the incremental validity of the *Common Factor* scores in predicting observed adolescent social anxiety, over and above individual informants' reports. In the first step of the regressions, individual informants' reports predicted observed adolescent social anxiety at small-to-large magnitudes. In the second step of the regressions, the *Common Factor* scores varied in the degree to which they displayed incremental validity, depending on the informant's report entered in the first step. Specifically, the *Common Factor* scores consistently explained incremental variance in observed adolescent social anxiety, over and above caregiver reports. In contrast, the *Common Factor* scores consistently failed to explain incremental variance, over and above peer confederate reports. Findings examining the incremental validity of the *Common Factor* score over and above adolescent reports were mixed. That is, whereas the three-informant *Common Factor* score explained incremental variance, the caregiver-adolescent *Common Factor* score did not. These findings indicate mixed support for the incremental validity of the *Common Factor* when predicting observed adolescent social anxiety.

We conducted hierarchical logistic regression analyses to determine the incremental validity of the *Common Factor* score in predicting adolescent referral status, over and above individual informants' reports. In the first step of the regressions, individual informants' reports predicted adolescent referral status. As with findings for observed social anxiety, in the second step of the regressions, the *Common Factor* scores varied in the degree to which they displayed incremental validity when predicting adolescent referral status, depending on the informant's report entered in the first step. Specifically, the caregiver-adolescent *Common Factor* score explained incremental variance over and above caregiver reports, and the adolescent-peer *Common Factor* explained incremental variance over and above peer confederate reports. In contrast, the adolescent-peer and caregiver-adolescent *Common Factor* scores failed to explain incremental variance in adolescent referral status,

Table 7.10 Hierarchical regressions examining the criterion-related validity of the Trifactor Model Common Factor score in predicting observed adolescent social anxiety relative to individual informants' reports (Study 2)

Step 1: Individual informants' report (caregiver) $\Delta R^2 = 0.05$, $\Delta F(1, 132) = 6.58$*		*Step 1*: Individual informants' report (adolescent) $\Delta R^2 = 0.22$, $\Delta F(1, 132) = 36.88$***		*Step 1*: Individual informants' report (peer confederate) $\Delta R^2 = 0.30$, $\Delta F(1, 128) = 53.89$***	
Variable	***B***	**Variable**	***B***	**Variable**	***B***
SPAIC	0.22*	**SPAIC**	0.47***	**SIAS**	0.54***
Step 2: Common Factor (adolescent-peer Trifactor Model) n/a		*Step 2*: Common Factor (adolescent-peer Trifactor Model) $\Delta R^2 = 0.002$, $\Delta F(1, 128) = 0.26$		*Step 2*: Common Factor (adolescent-peer Trifactor Model) $\Delta R^2 = 0.02$, $\Delta F(1, 127) = 2.81$	
Variable	***B***	**Variable**	***B***	**Variable**	***B***
–	–	**SPAIC**	0.42**	**SIAS**	0.47***
–	–	**Common Factor**	0.06	**Common Factor**	0.14
Step 2: Common Factor (caregiver-adolescent Trifactor Model) $\Delta R^2 = 0.11$, $\Delta F(1, 131) = 16.60$***		*Step 2*: Common Factor (caregiver-adolescent Trifactor Model) $\Delta R^2 = 0.002$, $\Delta F(1, 131) = 0.26$		*Step 2*: Common Factor (caregiver-adolescent Trifactor Model) n/a	
Variable	***B***	**Variable**	***B***	**Variable**	***B***
SPAIC	0.13	**SPAIC**	0.42***	–	–
Common Factor	0.34***	**Common Factor**	0.06	–	–
Step 2: Common Factor (3 informants) $\Delta R^2 = 0.12$, $\Delta F(1, 128) = 18.79$***		*Step 2*: Common Factor (3 informants) $\Delta R^2 = 0.06$, $\Delta F(1, 128) = 10.56$**		*Step 2*: Common Factor (3 informants) $\Delta R^2 = 0.001$, $\Delta F(1, 127) = 0.23$	
Variable	***B***	**Variable**	***B***	**Variable**	***B***
SPAIC	0.19*	**SPAIC**	0.40***	**SIAS**	0.58***
Common Factor	0.35***	**Common Factor**	0.25**	**Common Factor**	−0.05

Note: *SPAIC* Social Phobia and Anxiety Inventory for Children, *SIAS* Social Interaction Anxiety Scale; *$p < 0.05$; **$p < 0.01$; ***$p < 0.001$

over and above adolescent reports. The three-informant *Common Factor* score failed to explain incremental variance in adolescent referral status.

7.2.4.2 Incremental Validity of Scores Derived from the Trifactor Model Relative to the Composite Score (Tables 7.12 and 7.13)

We conducted a series of hierarchical linear regression models to evaluate whether the *Common Factor* scores explained variance in observed adolescent social anxiety, over and above the explanatory value of the SIAS composite score. In the first step of each regression model, the SIAS composite score explained significant variance in observed adolescent social anxiety, representing large effects. In the second

Table 7.11 Hierarchical regressions examining the criterion-related validity of the Trifactor Model Common Factor score in predicting referral status relative to individual informants' reports (Study 2)

Step 1: Individual informants' report (caregiver)		*Step 1*: Individual informants' report (adolescent)		*Step 1*: Individual informants' report (peer confederate)	
Variable	***OR***	**Variable**	***OR***	**Variable**	***OR***
SPAIC	1.10***	**SPAIC**	1.08***	**SIAS**	1.03*
Step 2: Common Factor (adolescent-peer Trifactor Model) n/a		*Step 2*: Common Factor (adolescent-peer Trifactor Model)		*Step 2*: Common Factor (adolescent-peer Trifactor Model)	
Variable	***OR***	**Variable**	***OR***	**Variable**	***OR***
–	–	**SPAIC**	1.06	**SIAS**	1.01
–	–	**Common Factor**	1.38	**Common Factor**	1.98**
Step 2: Common Factor (caregiver-adolescent Trifactor Model)		*Step 2*: Common Factor (caregiver-adolescent Trifactor Model)		*Step 2*: Common Factor (caregiver-adolescent Trifactor Model) n/a	
Variable	***OR***	**Variable**	***OR***	**Variable**	***OR***
SPAIC	1.09***	**SPAIC**	1.06*	–	–
Common Factor	1.99**	**Common Factor**	1.46	–	–
Step 2: Common Factor (3 informants)		*Step 2*: Common Factor (3 informants)		*Step 2*: Common Factor (3 informants)	
Variable	***OR***	**Variable**	***OR***	**Variable**	***OR***
SPAIC	1.10***	**SPAIC**	1.08***	**SIAS**	1.03
Common Factor	1.00	**Common Factor**	1.15	**Common Factor**	0.99

Note: *SPAIC* Social Phobia and Anxiety Inventory for Children, *SIAS* Social Interaction Anxiety Scale, *OR* Odds Ratio; *$p < 0.05$; **$p < 0.01$; ***$p < 0.001$

Table 7.12 Hierarchical regressions examining the criterion-related validity of the Trifactor Model Common Factor score in predicting observed adolescent social anxiety relative to the composite score approach (Study 2)

Step 1: Composite score (adolescent-peer reports) $\Delta R^2 = 0.34$, $\Delta F(1, 129) = 66.05$***		*Step 1*: Composite score (caregiver-adolescent reports) $\Delta R^2 = 0.23$, $\Delta F(1, 132) = 38.87$***		*Step 1*: Composite score (3 informants' reports) $\Delta R^2 = 0.34$, $\Delta F(1, 129) = 66.51$***	
Variable	***B***	**Variable**	***B***	**Variable**	***B***
Composite score	0.58***	**Composite score**	0.48***	**Composite score**	0.58***
Step 2: Common Factor (adolescent-peer Trifactor Model) $\Delta R^2 = 0.01$, $\Delta F(1, 128) = 1.59$		*Step 2*: Common Factor (caregiver-adolescent Trifactor Model) $\Delta R^2 = 0.01$, $\Delta F(1, 131) = 1.03$		*Step 2*: Common Factor (3 informants) $\Delta R^2 = 0.01$, $\Delta F(1, 128) = 1.30$	
Variable	***B***	**Variable**	***B***	**Variable**	***B***
Composite score	0.68***	**Composite score**	0.41***	**Composite score**	0.54***
Common Factor	−0.14	**Common Factor**	0.10	**Common Factor**	0.09

Note: *$p < 0.05$; **$p < 0.01$; ***$p < 0.001$

Table 7.13 Hierarchical regressions examining the criterion-related validity of the Trifactor Model Common Factor score in predicting referral status relative to the composite score approach (Study 2)

Step 1: Composite score (adolescent-peer reports)		*Step 1*: Composite score (caregiver-adolescent reports)		*Step 1*: Composite score (3 informants' reports)	
Variable	***OR***	**Variable**	***OR***	**Variable**	***OR***
Composite score	1.12***	**Composite score**	1.06***	**Composite score**	1.10***
Step 2: Common Factor (adolescent-peer Trifactor Model)		*Step 2*: Common Factor (caregiver-adolescent Trifactor Model)		*Step 2*: Common Factor (3 informants' reports)	
Variable	***OR***	**Variable**	***OR***	**Variable**	***OR***
Composite score	1.21***	**Composite score**	1.04	**Composite score**	1.12***
Common Factor	0.95	**Common Factor**	1.41	**Common Factor**	0.68

Note: *OR* Odds Ratio; $*p < 0.05$; $**p < 0.01$; $***p < 0.001$

step of each regression model, the *Common Factor* score did not explain incremental variance in observed adolescent social anxiety, over and above the SIAS composite score.

We also conducted a series of hierarchical logistic regression models to determine the incremental validity of the *Common Factor* score in predicting adolescent referral status, over and above the SIAS composite score. In the first step of each regression model, the SIAS composite score explained significant variance in adolescent referral status. In the second step of each regression model, the *Common Factor* score did not explain incremental variance in adolescent referral status, over and above the SIAS composite score.

7.2.4.3 Incremental Validity of the Satellite Model Trait Score Relative to Individual Informants' Reports (Tables 7.14 and 7.15)

We conducted hierarchical regression analyses to determine the incremental validity of the Satellite Model *Trait* score in predicting observed adolescent social anxiety, over and above individual informants' reports of social anxiety. In the first step of the regressions, individual informants' reports predicted observed adolescent social anxiety at moderate-to-large magnitudes. In the second step of the regressions, the *Trait* score consistently predicted incremental variance in observed adolescent social anxiety, over and above the variance explained by individual informants' reports, representing moderate-to-large effects.

We conducted hierarchical logistic regression analyses to determine the incremental validity of the *Trait* score in predicting adolescent referral status, over and above individual informants' reports of social anxiety. In the first step of the regressions, caregiver and adolescent reports predicted adolescent referral status, whereas peer confederate reports did not. As with findings for observed social anxiety, in the second step of the regressions, the *Trait* score predicted incremental variance in adolescent referral status, over and above the variance explained by individual

Table 7.14 Hierarchical regressions examining the criterion-related validity of the Satellite Model trait score in predicting observed adolescent social anxiety relative to individual informants' reports (Study 2)

Step 1: Individual informants' report (caregiver) $\Delta R^2 = 0.06$, $\Delta F(1, 130) = 7.73$**		*Step 1*: Individual informants' report (adolescent) $\Delta R^2 = 0.22$, $\Delta F(1, 130) = 35.70$***		*Step 1*: Individual informants' report (peer confederate) $\Delta R^2 = 0.24$, $\Delta F(1, 128) = 39.22$***	
Variable	***B***	**Variable**	***B***	**Variable**	***B***
SPAIC	0.24**	**SPAIC**	0.46***	**SPS**	0.48***
Step 2: Trait score $\Delta R^2 = 0.32$, $\Delta F(1, 129) = 65.59$***		*Step 2*: Trait score $\Delta R^2 = 0.14$, $\Delta F(1, 129) = 27.88$***		*Step 2*: Trait score $\Delta R^2 = 0.13$, $\Delta F(1, 127) = 26.63$***	
Variable	***B***	**Variable**	***B***	**Variable**	***B***
SPAIC	−0.18*	**SPAIC**	0.05	**SPS**	0.18*
Trait score	0.70***	**Trait score**	0.56***	**Trait score**	0.47***

Note: *SPAIC* Social Phobia and Anxiety Inventory for Children, *SPS* Social Phobia Scale; *$p < 0.05$; **$p < 0.01$; ***$p < 0.001$

Table 7.15 Hierarchical regressions examining the criterion-related validity of the Satellite Model trait score in predicting referral status relative to individual informants' reports (Study 2)

Step 1: Individual informants' report (caregiver)		*Step 1*: Individual informants' report (adolescent)		*Step 1*: Individual informants' report (peer confederate)	
Variable	***OR***	**Variable**	***OR***	**Variable**	***OR***
SPAIC	1.11**	**SPAIC**	1.08**	**SPS**	1.02
Step 2: Trait score		*Step 2*: Trait score		*Step 2*: Trait score	
Variable	***OR***	**Variable**	***OR***	**Variable**	***OR***
SPAIC	1.06	**SPAIC**	1.00	**SPS**	0.95
Trait score	2.64*	**Trait score**	3.50**	**Trait score**	6.83**

Note: *SPAIC* Social Phobia and Anxiety Inventory for Children, *SPS* Social Phobia Scale, *OR* Odds Ratio; *$p < 0.01$; **$p < 0.001$

informants' reports. Specifically, adolescents were three to seven times more likely to be clinic-referred (i.e., relative to community control), for every one-unit increase in the *Trait* score.

7.2.4.4 Incremental Validity of the Satellite Model Trait Score Relative to the Composite Score (Tables 7.16 and 7.17)

We conducted a hierarchical linear regression model to evaluate whether the Satellite Model *Trait* score explained variance in observed adolescent social anxiety, over and above the explanatory value of the composite score (i.e., average of caregiver, adolescent, and peer confederate SPS reports). In the first step of the regression, the composite score predicted observed adolescent social anxiety, representing a large effect. In the second step of the regression, the *Trait* score explained incremental variance in observed adolescent social anxiety, also representing a large effect.

Table 7.16 Hierarchical regressions examining the criterion-related validity of the Satellite Model trait score in predicting observed adolescent social anxiety relative to the composite score approach (Study 2)

Step 1: Composite score $\Delta R^2 = 0.28$, $\Delta F(1, 130) = 50.50^*$	
Variable	***B***
Composite score	0.53*
Step 2: Trait score $\Delta R^2 = 0.07$, $\Delta F\,(1, 129) = 14.80^*$	
Variable	***B***
Composite score	0.04
Trait score	0.56*

Note: *SPAIC* Social Phobia and Anxiety Inventory for Children, *SPS* Social Phobia Scale; $^*p < 0.001$

Table 7.17 Hierarchical regressions examining the criterion-related validity of the Satellite Model Trait score in predicting referral status relative to the composite score approach (Study 2)

Step 1: Composite score	
Variable	***OR***
Composite score	1.09**
Step 2: Trait score	
Variable	***OR***
Composite score	0.97
Trait score	5.18*

Note: *OR* Odds Ratio; $^*p < 0.01$; $^{**}p < 0.001$

We conducted a hierarchical logistic regression model to determine the incremental validity of the *Trait* score in predicting adolescent referral status, over and above the composite score. In the first step of the regression, the composite score predicted adolescent referral status. In the second step of the regression, the *Trait* score explained incremental variance in adolescent referral status. Adolescents were over five times more likely to be clinic-referred (i.e., relative to community control), for every one-unit increase in the *Trait* score.

7.2.5 *Aim 4: Directly Comparing the Incremental Validity of Scores Derived from the Trifactor Model and Satellite Model*

7.2.5.1 Preliminary Analyses

To compare the integrative scores obtained from the Trifactor Model and the Satellite Model, we conducted bivariate correlation analyses between the *Common Factor* and *Trait* scores using all three informants' reports. These analyses revealed a large-magnitude correlation between the *Common Factor* and *Trait* scores, $r = 0.50$, $p < 0.001$. Thus, these two integrative scores, which were derived from the same informants' reports on two distinct social anxiety measures, contained a fair degree of common variance yet also a fair degree of unique variance.

7.2.5.2 Incremental Validity of Scores Derived from the Satellite Model and Trifactor Model, Relative to Each Other

We conducted hierarchical linear regression models to evaluate whether the Trifactor Model *Common Factor* score explained variance in observed adolescent social anxiety, over and above the explanatory value of the Satellite Model *Trait* score and vice versa. We first evaluated the incremental validity of the *Common Factor* score. In the first step of the regression model, the *Trait* score explained significant variance in observed adolescent social anxiety, $\beta = 0.59$, $\Delta R^2 = 0.35$, $\Delta F(1, 128) = 68.11$, $p < 0.001$. In the second step of the regression model, the *Common Factor* score did not explain incremental variance in observed adolescent social anxiety, over and above the *Trait* score, $\beta = 0.08$, $\Delta R^2 = 0.01$, $\Delta F(1, 127) = 1.04$, $p = 0.31$. Next, we evaluated the incremental validity of the *Trait* score. In the first step of the regression model, the *Common Factor* score explained significant variance in observed adolescent social anxiety, $\beta = 0.36$, $\Delta R^2 = 0.13$, $\Delta F(1, 128) = 18.75$, $p < 0.001$. In the second step of the regression model, the *Trait* score explained incremental variance in observed adolescent social anxiety, over and above the *Common Factor* score, $\beta = 0.55$, $\Delta R^2 = 0.23$, $\Delta F(1, 127) = 44.12$, $p < 0.001$. Further, the *Common Factor* score no longer explained significant variance in observed adolescent social anxiety in the second step of the regression, $\beta = 0.08$, $p = 0.31$.

We conducted hierarchical logistic regression models to evaluate whether the *Common Factor* score explained variance in adolescent referral status, over and above the explanatory value of the *Trait* score and vice versa. We first evaluated the incremental validity of the *Common Factor* score. In the first step of the regression model, the *Trait* score explained significant variance in adolescent referral status, $b = 1.28$, $OR = 3.59$, $p < 0.001$. In the second step of the regression model, the *Common Factor* score did not explain incremental variance in adolescent referral status, over and above the *Trait* score, $b = -0.41$, $OR = 0.67$, $p = 0.13$. Next, we evaluated the incremental validity of the *Trait* score. In the first step of the regression model, the *Common Factor* score did not explain significant variance in adolescent referral status, $b = 0.35$, $OR = 1.42$, $p = 0.09$. In the second step of the regression model, the *Trait* score explained incremental variance in adolescent referral status, over and above the *Common Factor* score, $b = 1.51$, $OR = 4.54$, $p < 0.001$.

7.3 Concluding Comments

In sum, in Study 2, we found clear answers regarding the validity of scores derived from the Satellite Model and the Trifactor Model, relative to each other. Within data conditions in which discrepant results contain domain-relevant data, the Satellite

Model appears to offer an effective strategy for integrating informants' reports. In contrast, we observed mixed support for the criterion-related validity of *Common Factor* scores taken from the Trifactor Model. Specifically, the three-informant *Common Factor* score predicted observed adolescent social anxiety, representing a moderate effect, yet did not distinguish clinic-referred from community-control adolescents. The latter finding is particularly surprising given that in all but one instance, individual informants' reports predicted adolescents' referral status. This finding suggests that the Trifactor Model failed to incrementally predict domain-relevant criterion variables that individual informants could predict on their own.

Across Trifactor Models, *Common Factor* scores inconsistently predicted observed adolescent social anxiety and referral status, over and above individual informants' reports. These mixed findings are easily interpreted when considering each informants' factor loadings onto the *Common Factors* across Trifactor Models. We observed factor loadings for caregivers' reports at near-zero or relatively smaller magnitudes compared to other informants' loadings onto the *Common Factor*. Given this lack of overlapping variance, it is unsurprising that *Common Factor* scores predicted unique variance in observed behavior (and not referral status), over and above caregiver reports. In contrast, peer confederates' reports exhibited significant factor loadings in Trifactor Models, and thus, the *Common Factor* score did not provide incremental variance over and above the peer confederate reports. Importantly, both the individual peer confederate reports and caregiver reports displayed significant relations with the criterion variable. Thus, *Common Factor* scores performed no better in these models than an individual informant whose report displayed significant loadings onto the *Common Factor* and whose report displayed significant relations with the criterion variable. This is perhaps due to the assumption that variance shared among multiple informants' reports ought to outperform unique variance from an individual informant's report. Within data conditions that violate these assumptions (e.g., unique variance from informants contains valid information), *Common Factor* scores appear to hold little incremental value relative to reports from individual informants.

The inability of the *Common Factor* to predict independent criterion variables over and above the composite score also answers important questions about the validity of scores taken from the Trifactor Model. That is, although these two integrative strategies overlap in their emphasis on leveraging common variance to remove measurement confounds, the Trifactor Model is unique in its inclusion of a caregiver predictor thought to remove caregivers' "depressive bias." Thus, these findings suggest that removing this variance may actually detract from, instead of enhance, the validity of the scores taken from informants' reports. Within data conditions in which discrepant results contain domain-relevant data, the association between caregivers' own depressive symptoms and the unique information they provide when making reports about youth mental health is likely best explained by numerous domain-relevant features of family relationships, including environmental and genetic factors that increase risk for the development of youth psychopathology (e.g., Caspi et al., 2004; Goodman et al., 2020; Lindhiem et al., 2020).

References

Achenbach, T. M., McConaughy, S. H., & Howell, C. T. (1987). Child/adolescent behavioral and emotional problems: Implications of cross-informant correlations for situational specificity. *Psychological Bulletin, 101*(2), 213–232. https://psycnet.apa.org/doi/10.1037/0033-2909.101.2.213

Alfano, C. A., & Beidel, D. C. (2011). *Social anxiety in adolescents and young adults: Translating developmental science into practice*. American Psychological Association.

Armstrong, R. A. (2014). When to use the Bonferroni correction. *Ophthalmic and Physiological Optics, 34*(5), 502–508. https://doi.org/10.1111/opo.12131

Bartlett, M. S. (1950). Tests of significance in factor analysis. *British Journal of Psychology, 3*(2), 77–85. https://doi.org/10.1111/j.2044-8317.1950.tb00285.x

Bauer, D. J., Howard, A. L., Baldasaro, R. E., Curran, P. J., Hussong, A. M., Chassin, L., & Zucker, R. A. (2013). A trifactor model for integrating ratings across multiple informants. *Psychological Methods, 18*(4), 475–493. https://psycnet.apa.org/doi/10.1037/a0032475

Bentler, P. M. (1990). Comparative fit indexes in structural models. *Psychological Bulletin, 107*(2), 238–246. https://psycnet.apa.org/doi/10.1037/0033-2909.107.2.238

Cannon, C. J., Makol, B. A., Keeley, L. M., Qasmieh, N., Okuno, H., Racz, S. J., & De Los Reyes, A. (2020). A paradigm for understanding adolescent social anxiety with unfamiliar peers: Conceptual foundations and directions for future research. *Clinical Child and Family Psychology Review, 23*(3), 338–364. https://doi.org/10.1007/s10567-020-00314-4

Caspi, A., Moffitt, T. E., Morgan, J., Rutter, M., Taylor, A., Arseneault, L., et al. (2004). Maternal expressed emotion predicts children's antisocial behavior problems: Using monozygotic-twin differences to identify environmental effects on behavioral development. *Developmental Psychology, 40*(2), 149–161. https://psycnet.apa.org/doi/10.1037/0012-1649.40.2.149

Charamut, N. R., Racz, S. J., Wang, M., & De Los Reyes, A. (2022). Integrating multi-informant reports of youth mental health: A construct validation test of Kraemer and colleagues' (2003) satellite model. *Frontiers in Psychology, 13*, 911629. https://doi.org/10.3389/fpsyg.2022.911629

Clark, D. A., Durbin, C. E., Donnellan, M. B., & Neppl, T. K. (2017). Internalizing symptoms and personality traits color parental reports of child temperament. *Journal of Personality, 85*(6), 852–866. https://doi.org/10.1111/jopy.12293

Cohen, J. (1988). *Statistical power analysis for the behavioral sciences* (2nd ed.). Erlbaum.

Curran, P. J., Georgeson, A. R., Bauer, D. J., & Hussong, A. M. (2020). Psychometric models for scoring multiple reporter assessments: Applications to integrative data analysis in prevention science and beyond. *International Journal of Behavioral Development, 45*(1), 40–50. https://doi.org/10.1177/0165025419896620

De Los Reyes, A., Augenstein, T. M., Wang, M., Thomas, S. A., Drabick, D. A. G., Burgers, D., & Rabinowitz, J. (2015). The validity of the multi-informant approach to assessing child and adolescent mental health. *Psychological Bulletin, 141*(4), 858–900. https://doi.org/10.1037/a0038498

Deros, D. E., Racz, S. J., Lipton, M. F., Augenstein, T. M., Karp, J. N., Keeley, L. M., et al. (2018). Multi-informant assessments of adolescent social anxiety: Adding clarity by leveraging reports from unfamiliar peer confederates. *Behavior Therapy, 49*(1), 84–98. https://doi.org/10.1016/j.beth.2017.05.001

Etkin, R. G., Lebowitz, E. R., & Silverman, W. K. (2021a). Using evaluative criteria to review youth anxiety measures, part II: Parent-report. *Journal of Clinical Child and Adolescent Psychology, 50*(2), 155–176. https://doi.org/10.1080/15374416.2021.1878898

Etkin, R. G., Shimshoni, Y., Lebowitz, E. R., & Silverman, W. K. (2021b). Using evaluative criteria to review youth anxiety measures, part I: Self-report. *Journal of Clinical Child and Adolescent Psychology, 50*(1), 58–76. https://doi.org/10.1080/15374416.2020.1802736

Garb, H. N. (2003). Incremental validity and the assessment of psychopathology in adults. *Psychological Assessment, 15*(4), 508–520. https://doi.org/10.1037/1040-3590.15.4.508

Glenn, L. E., Keeley, L. M., Szollos, S., Okuno, H., Wang, X., Rausch, E., Deros, D. E., Karp, J. N., Qasmieh, N., Makol, B. A., Augenstein, T. M., Lipton, M. F., Racz, S. J., Scharfstein, L., Beidel, D. C., & De Los Reyes, A. (2019). Trained observers' ratings of adolescents' social anxiety and social skills within controlled, cross-contextual social interactions with unfamiliar peer confederates. *Journal of Psychopathology and Behavioral Assessment, 41*(1), 1–15. https://doi.org/10.1007/s10862-018-9676-4

Goodman, S. H., Simon, H. F. M., Shamblaw, A. L., & Kim, C. Y. (2020). Parenting as a mediator of associations between depression in mothers and children's functioning: A systematic review and meta-analysis. *Clinical Child and Family Psychology Review, 23*(4), 427–460. https://doi.org/10.1007/s10567-020-00322-4

Hu, L., & Bentler, P. M. (1999). Cutoff criteria for fit indexes in covariance structure analysis: Conventional criteria versus new alternatives. *Structural Equation Modeling: A Multidisciplinary Journal, 6*(1), 1–55. https://doi.org/10.1080/10705519909540118

Hunsley, J., & Meyer, G. J. (2003). The incremental validity of psychological testing and assessment: Conceptual, methodological, and statistical issues. *Psychological Assessment, 15*(4), 446–455. https://doi.org/10.1037/1040-3590.15.4.446

Kaiser, H. F. (1970). A second generation little jiffy. *Psychometrika, 35*(4), 401–415. https://psycnet.apa.org/doi/10.1007/BF02291817

Keeley, L. M., Laird, R. D., Qasmieh, N., Racz, S. J., Ohannessian, C. M., & De Los Reyes, A. (2024). When parents and adolescents make discrepant reports about parental monitoring: Links to adolescent anxiety when interacting with unfamiliar peers. *Journal of Psychopathology and Behavioral Assessment, 46*(2), 343–356. https://doi.org/10.1007/s10862-024-10132-5

Kline, R. B. (2016). *Principles and practice of structural equation modeling* (4th ed.). Guilford.

Kraemer, H. C., Measelle, J. R., Ablow, J. C., Essex, M. J., Boyce, W. T., & Kupfer, D. J. (2003). A new approach to integrating data from multiple informants in psychiatric assessment and research: Mixing and matching contexts and perspectives. *American Journal of Psychiatry, 160*(9), 1566–1577. https://doi.org/10.1176/appi.ajp.160.9.1566

Lindhiem, O., Vaughn-Coaxum, R. A., Higa, J., Harris, J. L., Kolko, D. J., & Pilkonis, P. A. (2020). Development and validation of the Parenting Skill Use Diary (PSUD) in a nationally representative sample. *Journal of Clinical Child and Adolescent Psychology, 50*(3), 400–410. https://doi.org/10.1080/15374416.2020.1716366

Makol, B. A. (2022). *Bias versus context models for integrating multi-informant reports of youth mental health* (order no. 28547966). Available from ProQuest Dissertations & Theses Global. (2718669547). https://www.proquest.com/dissertations-theses/bias-versus- context-models-integrating-multi/docview/2718669547/se-2

Makol, B. A., Youngstrom, E. A., Racz, S. J., Qasmieh, N., Glenn, L. E., & De Los Reyes, A. (2020). Integrating multiple informants' reports: How conceptual and measurement models may address long-standing problems in clinical decision-making. *Clinical Psychological Science, 8*(6), 953–970. https://doi.org/10.1177/2167702620924439

Martel, M. M., Markon, K., & Smith, G. T. (2017a). Research review: Multi-informant integration in child and adolescent psychopathology diagnosis. *Journal of Child Psychology and Psychiatry, 58*(2), 116–128. https://doi.org/10.1111/jcpp.12611

Martel, M. M., Nigg, J. T., & Schimmack, U. (2017b). Psychometrically informed approach to integration of multiple informant ratings in adult ADHD in a community-recruited sample. *Assessment, 24*(3), 279–289. https://doi.org/10.1177/1073191116646443

McDonald, R. P., & Ho, M. H. R. (2002). Principles and practice in reporting structural equation analyses. *Psychological Methods, 7*(1), 64–82. https://doi.org/10.1037/1082-989X.7.1.64

Pett, M. A., Lackey, N. R., & Sullivan, J. J. (2003). *Making sense of factor analysis: The use of factor analysis for instrument development in health care research*. Sage.

Richters, J. E. (1992). Depressed mothers as informants about their children: A critical review of the evidence for distortion. *Psychological Bulletin, 112*(3), 485–499. https://doi.org/10.1037/0033-2909.112.3.485

Smith, G. T., Fischer, S., & Fister, S. M. (2003). Incremental validity principles in test construction. *Psychological Assessment, 15*(4), 467–477. https://doi.org/10.1037/1040-3590.15.4.467

Steiger, J. H. (1990). Structural model evaluation and modification: An interval estimation approach. *Multivariate Behavioral Research, 25*(2), 173–180. https://doi.org/10.1207/s15327906mbr2502_4

Streiner, D. L., & Norman, G. R. (2011). Correction for multiple testing: Is there a resolution? *Chest, 140*(1), 16–18. https://doi.org/10.1378/chest.11-0523

Tucker, L. R., & Lewis, C. (1973). A reliability coefficient for maximum likelihood factor analysis. *Psychometrika, 38*(1), 1–10. https://doi.org/10.1007/BF02291170

Chapter 8
Decision-Making About Strategies for Integrating Behavioral Data in Youth Development

Scholars in youth development conduct studies that entail collecting and interpreting reports from structurally different informants (e.g., parents, teachers, youth, peers). Structurally different informants are strategically selected informants. That is, scholars choose informants who each contribute unique and incrementally valid information. When assessing youth behavior, this means selecting informants who observe behavior in domain-relevant contexts. Decades of research and meta-analytic reviews reveal that the use of structurally different informants produces discrepancies between informants' reports (De Los Reyes, 2024). These discrepancies impact decision-making across a range of research and applied settings (De Los Reyes et al., 2022a, b). Logically, discrepant results necessitate the use of strategies for integrating data. Yet there exist no evidence-based guidelines for which integrative strategies to use and when to use them (e.g., De Los Reyes et al., 2023b; Hunsley & Mash, 2007). Relatedly, we see a lack of synergy among conceptual models, empirical support for these models, and attention to thoroughly examining the fit of strategies for integrating multi-informant data (e.g., De Los Reyes & Epkins, 2023). Among the available strategies, two stem from theoretical models that call for qualitatively distinct approaches to integrating data. Social context models are rooted in the concept of situational specificity (Achenbach et al., 1987). They call for integrative strategies such as the Satellite Model, which treat as potential sources of valid data (a) variance that is shared among informants' reports, but also (b) variance that is unique (i.e., as is reflected by discrepant results). In contrast, rater bias models, many of which are rooted in the depression→distortion hypothesis (Ritchers, 1992), call for integrative strategies such as the Trifactor Model, which treat common variance as the only source of valid data.

Informed by the Operations Triad Model and CONTEXT (De Los Reyes et al., 2023a)—a framework and associated validation paradigm designed for the data conditions encountered by scholars in youth development—this book addressed fundamental gaps in the evidence base on strategies for integrating data from structurally different informants. The findings from a multi-modal set of studies

B. A. Makol et al., *Youth Development in Context*, Springer Series on Child and Family Studies, https://doi.org/10.1007/978-3-031-80549-3_8

highlight how the theoretical model one follows when integrating multi-informant data guides all decisions within the assessment process, ranging from how users of these models select informants to how they obtain and interpret integrative scores. Across two studies, we learned that relative to scores derived from the Trifactor Model, scores derived from the Satellite Model display the most robust evidence in support of their criterion-related validity. Specifically, integrating multi-informant data using scores taken from the Satellite Model achieves more in prediction than any one informant can achieve on their own. The Satellite Model *Trait* score also outperformed a composite score of reports—a strategy one uses when assuming unique variance among reports reflects measurement confounds. Further, this score outperformed the Trifactor Model *Common Factor* score, which its developers contend reflects common variance that "purges" unique biases from individual informants' reports. When using three informants' reports, the Trifactor Model *Common Factor* score failed to consistently outperform individual informants' reports. The use of the *Common Factor* score reduced measurement validity in two ways. First, it reduced the incremental value of integrative scores, relative to individual reports and a composite score of reports. Second, features of the Trifactor Model that, in theory, partial out variance reflecting rater biases (i.e., *Perspective Factors*), in practice, led to removing valid data contained within informants' reports.

To be clear, decisions surrounding the strategy one implements to integrate multi-informant data do not rest on whether the Trifactor Model or Satellite Model are "correct strategies." Rather, users must judge for themselves whether a strategy validly fits the data conditions to which they will apply the strategy. The studies reported in this book align with calls for the use of well-established measurement validation procedures to determine the fit between integrative strategies and data conditions (see De Los Reyes, 2024; De Los Reyes et al., 2023a, b; Greene et al., 2022; Revelle, 2024). Our studies indicate that when discrepant results contain domain-relevant or valid data, users ought to leverage integrative strategies that treat these discrepancies as valid (e.g., Satellite Model). The take-home message of our findings is clear. In youth development—a community of scholars who often implement multi-informant approaches to collect behavioral data—negative consequences flow from violating the usage assumptions of strategies for integrating these data. In this community—and perhaps others—scholars should avoid the use of a strategy for integrating multi-informant data when the data conditions to which they might apply it violate the strategy's usage assumptions. A lack of fit between an integrative strategy and the data conditions to which it will be applied will lead to integrative scores with lower observed effect sizes and thus less statistical power to detect effects, relative to integrative strategies that do fit the data conditions. Within some data conditions, an ill-fitting integrative strategy may even "lose" to reports from the individual informants involved in the strategy.

8.1 Research and Applied Implications

8.1.1 What Is in a Name?

This book highlights a series of larger issues for scholars in youth development to consider. First, developers of integrative strategies often disseminate them to prospective users before testing how these models perform in relation to domain-relevant, independent criterion variables. This represents a serious barrier to building consensus guidelines on how and under what circumstances to integrate multi-informant data. The most common data used to support integrative strategies are fit indices as well as factor and component loadings (Greene et al., 2022). These are useful indicators of model precision. Yet they cannot fully address how integrative strategies perform when scholars put the scores these strategies produce "to the test." Scholars who seek guidance on strategies for integrating multi-informant data—and for use in studies that address practical problems of societal relevance—need more than estimates of model precision to make accurate and informed decisions (see also Revelle, 2024). They also need carefully conducted multi-modal tests of measurement validity. These tests allow users to tease apart the variance produced by integrative strategies that reflect "junk" from the variance that reflects "real stuff" (see also De Los Reyes, 2024; Talbott et al., 2023; Watts et al., 2022).

This book addresses questions about the criterion-related validity of integrative strategies such as the Trifactor Model and the Satellite Model. More broadly, this book reveals a paradigm for scrutinizing, testing, and using analytic strategies, particularly when they vary as to their usage assumptions. For example, a key issue surrounding the use of the Trifactor Model and the Satellite Model is how model developers approached interpreting scores derived from these models. The researchers who developed these models are both guilty of the "naming fallacy" (Kline, 2016), whereby they interpreted the meaning of measured factors without the use of valid evidence to support their interpretations. Consequently, in Study 2, we used independent criterion variables to determine whether the key integrative scores derived from the Trifactor Model and the Satellite Model (i.e., *Common Factor* and *Trait*, respectively) validly characterized the behavioral domain about which informants made reports (i.e., adolescent social anxiety). Future research using other criterion variables is needed to fully unpack the interpretive value of scores derived from the Trifactor Model and Satellite Model, such as independent assessments of caregiver mood and observed interactions between adolescents and caregivers.

That said, Study 2 findings suggest that when implemented within data conditions that contain domain-relevant discrepant results, it would be incorrect to interpret the *Perspective Factors* in line with the interpretation provided by its developers. Following Bauer and colleagues' interpretation of the caregiver *Perspective Factor*, one would essentially remove variance attributed to caregivers' reports under the assumption that it reflects a rater bias, even within data conditions in which this variance meaningfully relates to domain-relevant criterion variables. By construction, measurement confounds reflect irrelevant variance—they should be unrelated to indices that reflect domain-relevant phenomena (see Millsap, 2011). What this means is that within data conditions in which users detect links between the *Perspective Factor* and independent, domain-relevant criterion variables, such an observation should give users pause as to whether the Trifactor Model is appropriate to implement as designed. We must critically examine integrative scores to unpack the type of information they contain (i.e., measurement confounds vs. domain-relevant data) and evaluate their ability to characterize youth behavior. More broadly, we must question not only what is gained from leveraging scores taken from integrative strategies, but also what is lost. These questions can be readily addressed by subjecting scores taken from integrative strategies to well-constructed validation tests.

8.1.2 What Do We Lose When Integrative Strategies Compete with One Another?

The Satellite Model and the Trifactor Model grew out of distinct theoretical traditions. We presume that they reflect competing strategies for integrating multi-informant reports. Yet, must they compete? This book subjected two integrative strategies to a head-to-head competition for explaining variance in domain-relevant outcomes. This approach yielded some key insights as to the value of these two strategies, given the set of data conditions to which they were applied. That said, our approach to validation testing is not without its drawbacks. We see three issues arising when scholars pit competing integrative strategies against one another.

First, might such an approach result in losing sight of how strategies complement one another? Although a strong evidence base supports the notion that discrepant results often contain domain-relevant data, we should also keep in mind that any index of these discrepancies cannot be "perfect." It would be safe to assume that informants' reports tend to contain some degree of measurement confounds. It logically follows that at least some of these confounds "filter into" indices of the discrepancies between informants' reports (Borsboom 2005; Nunnally & Bernstein, 1994). Consequently, should we seek to create integrative strategies that model not only variance reflecting domain-relevant discrepant results, but also variance that reflects rater biases? To address this larger question, we must first conduct basic research focused on estimating the variance explained by both rater biases and domain-relevant processes. This knowledge might inform new integrative strategies. These strategies would allow users to extract measured scores that isolate variance attributable to rater biases and domain-relevant processes and subject these scores to both Monte Carlo simulations and well-constructed measurement validation tests to assess their performance. Importantly, the ability to model multiple sources of variance in discrepant results will not absolve researchers of the need for validation testing. Indeed, even if one were to discover evidence of rater biases in a study of youth behavior (e.g., depression-distortion effects), this factor might account for relatively little variation within and among informants' reports (e.g., see Jouriles & Thompson, 1993; Youngstrom et al., 1999).

Second, might our approach to testing competing integrative strategies result in acts of omission when it comes to detecting sources of rater bias? For instance, Study 2 revealed that when users of the Trifactor Model treat caregivers' depression as a source of rater bias—and it, in fact, reflects variability that meaningfully relates to youth behavior (i.e., is domain-relevant)—the result is a loss of valid data and, by extension, loss of explanatory power. Such an observation may compel at least some users of the Trifactor Model or alternative integrative strategies to assume that their efforts in detecting sources of rater bias are complete. This may be a mistake. Although the depression→distortion hypothesis is the most widely studied rater bias model, other rater bias models warrant further study. We must also subject these rater bias models to rigorous testing, including models that focus on racial biases (Fadus et al., 2020; Kang & Harvey, 2020) and cultural perspectives on youth behavior (Achenbach, 2020; Chen et al., 2017; Lau et al., 2004). We must probe the links between discrepant results and integrative strategies informed by rater bias models other than the depression→distortion hypothesis.

Third, in avoiding acts of omission regarding sources of rater biases, we must avoid acts of commission as well. As with the depression→distortion hypothesis, we must subject all rater bias models to scrutiny, particularly regarding their conceptual foundations and evidence base. Recall in Chap. 1 how we deconstructed the depression→distortion hypothesis and its core assumption—that all discrepant results reflect mood-congruent rater biases. Those who hold these presumably mood-congruent rater biases are significant others in the lives of the youth being assessed (e.g., caregivers). To posit that a significant other's mood levels reflect nothing more than a source of biased ratings ignores decades of scholarship in youth development—a body of work that finds that significant others' behavior affects youth behavior (Atkins et al., 2017; Carlone & Milan, 2021; Cicchetti, 1984; Goodman et al., 2020; Luthar et al., 2000).

Beyond the depression→distortion hypothesis, let us consider a rater bias model informed by scholarship about racial biases. Here, the rater bias model would be quite distinct from the rater bias model we focused on in this book. In a rater bias model linked to racial biases, increased levels of a characteristic of the informant (racial biases) would predict increased discrepant results in reports about the behavior of a target set of youth. For the purposes of this example, let us say the informants of interest are teachers, and the reports they provide focus on the behavior of students in teachers' classrooms. The discrepancies would be the byproduct of inaccuracies in teachers' perceptions not of all students, but rather students with specific characteristics. An example of these characteristics might be students who identify with racial groups that have been historically marginalized in a specific geographic region, such as the USA. A model that treats racial biases as sources of rater bias would characterize all the discrepant results in reports about youth who identify with historically marginalized groups as reflective of rater biases. In our example, these would be measurement confounds in teachers' reports linked to the racial biases they hold about students with specific racial identities (e.g., African American,

Asian American, Native American; see Hurd & Young, 2023; West et al., 2023). The key question is this: Would it be correct to treat all these discrepant results as measurement confounds? In this example, measurement confounds, by definition, would reflect variance that is irrelevant to understanding the behavior of the students who teachers rate. Yet teachers are not passive observers of students' behavior. They lead classrooms of students, and thus, how they behave impacts how students behave (see also Atkins et al., 2017). In scholarship in youth development, teachers can serve as raters of students' behavior and as catalysts of the very behaviors they rate. How a teacher perceives their students could be inaccurate. Yet this inaccurate perception can have a real-world impact on the behavior of the students they rate.

Consider a hypothetical version of our Study 2, in which we examined the reports of teachers as informants, the youth in the sample were students in their classrooms, and the validity criterion was an index of how youth behaved in class. In this study, we measured teachers' levels of racial biases and used this measure as our index of rater biases (i.e., as opposed to the use of caregivers' levels of depression as rater biases for the Trifactor Model tested in Study 2). What if we found the same pattern of findings as we did in Study 2? Specifically, we treated all the variance produced by the racial bias index as a "rater bias," but in doing so, we reduced the score validity of teachers' reports when predicting how youth behaved as measured by the validity criterion (e.g., classroom behavior). If teachers rate students' behavior and increased racial biases predict increased disparities in how teachers actually treat students of varying racial identities, then would we not expect teachers' behavior to, in turn, impact how students behave? This would be akin to the depression example: Would we be correct to assume that the racial biases that a teacher holds have no effect on the behavior of the youth with whom they interact? Would not this assumption run counter to decades of research and theory in youth development? This work finds that exposure to discriminatory racial encounters plays a role in the development and maintenance of such behaviors as aversive stress reactions and mental health concerns (e.g., Anderson & Stevenson, 2019; Price et al., 2022; Scott et al., 2021).

This discussion reveals a reality about scholarship. The term "bias" can create confusion among scholars if its meaning varies within and across scholarly traditions. Scholars who study psychometrics consider the term "bias" as synonymous with the term "measurement confounds" (e.g., De Los Reyes et al., 2022b, c; Millsap, 2011; Nunnally & Bernstein, 1994; Tabachnick & Fidell, 2013). In psychometrics, measurement confounds are data that are irrelevant to understanding measured domains. We can distinguish this use of "bias" from its use in contemporary scholarship on racism and discrimination. Scholars who study racism and discrimination consider biases to be both relevant and central to understanding human behavior. Future work on rater bias models must consider strategies for integrating distinct scholarly traditions and approaches to studying bias. This will necessitate developing conceptual and empirical approaches that allow for the accurate decomposition of sources of variability that reflect measurement confounds and in a way that distinguishes these confounds from sources of variability that are pertinent to understanding behavior.

8.1.3 Implications for Decision-Making in Applied Settings

Our findings also have important implications for how users incorporate multi-informant data when making decisions in applied settings, such as clinics, schools, and legislative offices. For instance, we can see Compensating Operations reflected in the delivery of mental health services. It is common for assessors who encounter discrepant data from informants to choose the "optimal" informant or the source most likely to report the "truth" (see De Los Reyes et al., 2022a; Marsh et al., 2020). What this means is that just as a researcher may utilize a rater bias model, professionals in applied settings might collect multi-informant data to understand behavior, only to ignore some of these data if all informants fail to agree. As described by Etkin et al. (2021), taking a bias-aligned approach leads to professionals getting stuck in the "right-versus-wrong conundrum" when interpreting discrepant results (p. 157). One can clearly see the implications of this approach for a variety of decision-making scenarios, including selecting students for receipt of an educational program, and the consideration of evidence from multiple sources of data when making a policy decision.

In contrast, taking a CONTEXT-aligned approach facilitates testing hypotheses about why behavior may differ across relevant social contexts. Future work should leverage integrative strategies in applied settings and evaluate whether the use of these models enhances the accuracy of decision-making. Further, this work should probe the impact of these strategies on key outcomes. As an example, consider the value of this work for clinical practice settings. Future work might examine whether strategies vary in the prediction of therapeutic processes and the outcomes of the services youth receive. These findings have the potential to inform work on *measurement-based care*—the systematic and continuous assessment of mental health throughout treatment for the purpose of monitoring progress and informing clinical decision-making (see McLeod et al., 2022). For instance, future work should examine how integrative scores such as the *Trait* score can be normed in ways that are amenable to translation into interpretable feedback paradigms for both clinicians and youth (e.g., non-clinical, borderline, and clinical cutoffs; Achenbach, 2001). Yet, to be successful, these feedback paradigms must be sensitive to common barriers to implementing evidence-based assessment practices in routine clinical care (e.g., time and motivation for youth to complete measures, resistance by clinicians to use reports to inform decision-making, lack of resources provided by clinics to train clinicians on how to use reports, lack of funding for measures and computer programs for scoring them; Lewis et al., 2019).

Let us consider a set of clinical vignettes that illustrate how the use of rater bias and social context models leads to fundamentally different decision-making practices, to highlight the need for future work on these issues. Take for example a mother bringing her preschooler to therapy given concerns about the child's disruptive and oppositional behavior. The clinician administers symptom measures to the child's mother and teacher and finds that the mother reported very elevated levels of externalizing behaviors, whereas the teacher did not. Through a clinical interview, the clinician learns that the child's mother experienced depression over the past year, which has contributed to feelings of guilt about her parenting, fewer positive parent-child interactions, and inconsistent use of strategies to address the child's behavior. If the clinician draws from rater bias models, they may consider disregarding the mother's reports given concerns about a depressive bias that reduces the validity of her reports. The clinician may then turn to the teacher as an "unbiased" expert on the child's behavior who is better equipped to report the "truth." In doing so, the clinician may conclude that the child is not experiencing clinically significant mental health problems and the family would be best served through individual therapy for depression with the child's mother only. This decision, however, does not track with scholarship in youth mental health, in particular the robust link between caregiver mental health and the development and maintenance of the mental health of youth in their care (e.g., Carlone & Milan, 2021; Goodman et al., 2020). In essence, does this clinical decision serve the child in need of services, if the mother's depression reflects a feature of the youth's environment that may already be exhibiting a direct impact on the child's mental health?

Alternatively, if the clinician draws from social context models, they may develop hypotheses about where the child's problem behavior is occurring and environmental conditions and antecedents that promote and maintain the behavior. As identified by the child's mother, home may be characterized by high levels of criticism (as opposed to praise), inconsistent discipline, and poor parent-child attachment, risk factors associated with the development of mental health problems in early childhood and in the context of caregiver depression (Goodman et al., 2020; Lindhiem et al., 2020). The clinician can then consider how to target the child's behavior by reshaping the primary context in which the behavior is occurring, utilizing evidence-based interventions that promote positive parent-child interactions as well as effective and consistent use of discipline (e.g., Child-Parent Psychotherapy or Parent-Child Interaction Therapy; Lieberman et al., 2015; Eyberg & Funderberk, 2011).

As another example, consider a scenario in which a family is seeking an ADHD evaluation for their adolescent daughter. The assessor collects symptom reports from the adolescent's father and teacher, as well as the adolescent herself. The assessor finds that all informants converge in elevated ADHD symptom reports. Yet, whereas the adolescent reports moderate levels of anxiety, her father reports no anxiety concerns, and her teacher reports elevated anxiety concerns as well as depressive symptoms. If the assessor follows a rater bias model approach, they may consider bias in two forms. First, the adolescent's father may have a *social desirability bias* in which he wants to minimize the perception that his daughter struggles with anxiety (Rodriguez et al., 2019). Second, the teacher's report might be understood as suffering from an *evaluative consistency bias* in which the teacher inaccurately endorses a broad range of difficulties due to elevated concerns in only one domain (i.e., ADHD; Dhillon et al., 2017). When providing feedback to the family, the assessor can then consider communicating that either the father or teacher is "missing the mark" on anxiety due to biases contained in their ratings. Such an approach is likely to isolate information-gathering to just a single informant used within the evaluation. From a practical standpoint, this approach then begs the question: Why did the clinician select the father and teacher for the expert information they provide, only to deem their reports as fallible, presumably based on the discrepant results they produced?

Alternatively, if the assessor adopts a social context model approach, they may form hypotheses about aspects of the adolescent's social environments that elicit (or do not elicit) anxiety. In a clinical interview with the adolescent, the assessor may learn that the adolescent's ADHD symptoms are causing significant anxiety about academics particularly at school (e.g., ADHD-related impairment leads to low self-esteem and anxiety about academic failure). However, the adolescent may experience minimal anxiety at home due to regular organizational support and low levels of pressure from her caregivers on academic tasks (e.g., support on homework, regular praise about academic strengths). When providing feedback to the family, the assessor can encourage the caregivers to continue their supportive approach and recommend therapy for the adolescent to learn coping strategies to use at school to reduce anxiety (e.g., Cognitive Behavioral Therapy for ADHD; Sprich et al., 2016). Taken together, these clinical vignettes highlight how the act of taking a rater bias or social context model approach when interpreting assessment data in applied settings translates to fundamentally different decisions regarding decision-making and, in the case of clinical practice, the delivery of mental health services. As such, they highlight the need for future work that takes a measurement-based care approach to develop clinically feasible approaches to addressing discrepant results when working with youth.

8.2 Limitations

Findings reported in this book should be interpreted in light of the limitations of our studies. First, the two integrative strategies we evaluated are illustrative of strategies informed by rater bias or social context models about what discrepant results reflect. Yet they are not the only strategies available. As such, this study does not put to rest conceptual, empirical, or measurement issues that arise when collecting multi-informant reports, encountering discrepant results, and using strategies for integrating multi-informant data. The Satellite Model, Trifactor Model, and other strategies must undergo additional validation testing within many data conditions. A crucial next step would be to subject integrative strategies to both simulated and "real-world" data conditions in which the discrepant results produced reflect measurement confounds.

A limitation of Study 2 is the relatively small sample used to address aims. We selected the sample for its wide breadth of modalities (e.g., parallel informants' reports on multiple social anxiety measures, observed behavior) and the psychometric evidence supporting the use of these modalities (for a review, see De Los Reyes, 2024). Given the amount of resources required to collect these kinds of multi-modal assessment data, it is rare to find large datasets that include several informants' reports and independent, domain-relevant criterion variables. Nonetheless, future research should address similar aims in a dataset consisting of a larger sample. Relatedly, Study 2 lacked independent criterion variables capturing caregivers' mood as well as adolescent behavior within other salient contexts (e.g., home, classroom). Although our use of caregivers' self-reported mood is consistent with empirical studies examining the depression→distortion hypothesis and applications of the Trifactor Model (e.g., Curran et al., 2020; Madsen et al., 2020), this shared method variance between caregivers' self-reported depression and their reports of adolescent social anxiety creates issues with shared method variance among the reports used to estimate discrepant results and the reports used for covariates (see Garb, 2003; Watts et al., 2022).

Lastly, the mix-and-match criterion of the Satellite Model and informants available within our Study 2 sample prevented us from examining various informant triads in the Satellite Model. This is in contrast to modeling for the Trifactor Model, which included various informant dyads as well as an informant triad. Granted, informant triads beyond those tested in Study 2 have been implemented in prior work by multiple independent research teams (e.g., Armstrong et al., 2014; De Los Reyes et al., 2022c; Gardner et al., 2008; Owens & Hinshaw, 2016). Yet, as mentioned previously, little validation work has put this approach to the test with independent, domain-relevant criterion variables. Thus, future research should focus on identifying the range of informants appropriate for the Satellite Model.

8.3 Concluding Comments

Scholars in youth development frequently encounter discrepant results in assessments about youth behavior. These discrepancies necessitate sound strategies for integrating data commonly collected by scholars in youth development, namely, data from multi-informant assessments. Yet scholars lack consensus guidelines for integrating these data. Many integrative strategies have been proposed, and these strategies each fall within one of two distinct theoretical traditions (i.e., rater bias models vs. social context models). The assumptions underlying the use of strategies informed by these theoretical models are consequential and dictate the degree to which an integrative strategy produces scores that capitalize on the rich, contextually sensitive data produced by multi-informant assessments of youth behavior.

Across two studies, we learned that selecting strategies for integrating multi-informant data involves (a) developing a deep understanding of the data conditions to which they will be applied and (b) subjecting these strategies to the same kinds of validation tests that inform the development, selection, and implementation of instruments for assessing youth behavior. Within data conditions in which discrepant results contain domain-relevant data, the choice is clear. When discrepant results contain valid data, scholars should implement an integrative strategy that flows from a social context model, such as the Satellite Model.

This book is but a start to a larger body of work that addresses myriad questions relevant to scholarship in youth development. What do discrepant results reflect, and does the answer to this question depend on the behaviors scholars seek to assess? Within the data conditions that typify scholarship in youth development, what statistical approaches are most appropriate for integrating multi-informant data? Which approaches optimize the value of these data when making decisions within applied settings? Across these key questions, we require studies that strategically discern the fit among theoretical traditions, the integrative strategies that flow from them, and the data conditions to which strategies will be applied. Aligning these crucial elements within scholarly and applied work is the path most likely to advance knowledge about youth development and result in sound decision-making when working with data that frequently produce discrepant results about youth behavior.

References

Achenbach, T. M. (2001). *Child behavior checklist for ages 6 to 18*. University of Vermont Research Center for Children, Youth, and Families.

Achenbach, T. M. (2020). Bottom-up and top-down paradigms for psychopathology: A half century odyssey. *Annual Review of Clinical Psychology, 16*, 1–24. https://doi.org/10.1146/annurev-clinpsy-071119-115831

Achenbach, T. M., McConaughy, S. H., & Howell, C. T. (1987). Child/adolescent behavioral and emotional problems: Implications of cross-informant correlations for situational specificity. *Psychological Bulletin, 101*(2), 213–232. https://psycnet.apa.org/doi/10.1037/0033-2909.101.2.213

Anderson, R. E., & Stevenson, H. C. (2019). RECASTing racial stress and trauma: Theorizing the healing potential of racial socialization in families. *American Psychologist, 74*(1), 63–75. https://doi.org/10.1037/amp0000392

Armstrong, J. M., Ruttle, P. L., Klein, M. H., Essex, M. J., & Benca, R. M. (2014). Associations of child insomnia, sleep movement, and their persistence with mental health symptoms in childhood and adolescence. *Sleep, 37*(5), 901–909. https://psycnet.apa.org/doi/10.5665/sleep.3656

Atkins, M. S., Cappella, E., Shernoff, E. S., Mehta, T. G., & Gustafson, E. L. (2017). Schooling and children's mental health: Realigning resources to reduce disparities and advance public health. *Annual Review of Clinical Psychology, 13*, 123–147. https://doi.org/10.1146/annurev-clinpsy-032816-045234

Borsboom, D. (2005). *Measuring the mind*. Cambridge University Press.

Carlone, C., & Milan, S. (2021). Maternal depression and child externalizing behaviors: The role of attachment across development in low-income families. *Research on Child and Adolescent Psychopathology, 49*(5), 603–614. https://doi.org/10.1007/s10802-020-00747-z

Chen, Y. Y., Ho, S. Y., Lee, P. C., Wu, C. K., & Gau, S. S. F. (2017). Parent-child discrepancies in the report of adolescent emotional and behavioral problems in Taiwan. *PLoS One, 12*(6), e0178863. https://doi.org/10.1371/journal.pone.0178863

Cicchetti, D. (1984). The emergence of developmental psychopathology. *Child Development, 55*(1), 1–7. https://doi.org/10.2307/1129830

Curran, P. J., Georgeson, A. R., Bauer, D. J., & Hussong, A. M. (2020). Psychometric models for scoring multiple reporter assessments: Applications to integrative data analysis in prevention science and beyond. *International Journal of Behavioral Development, 45*(1), 40–50. https://doi.org/10.1177/0165025419896620

De Los Reyes, A. (2024). *Discrepant results in mental health research: What they mean, why they matter, and how they inform scientific practices*. Oxford University Press.

De Los Reyes, A., Cook, C. R., Sullivan, M., Morrell, N., Hamlin, C., Wang, M., Gresham, F. M., Makol, B. A., Keeley, L. M., & Qasmieh, N. (2022c). The Work and Social Adjustment Scale for Youth: Psychometric properties of the teacher version and evidence of contextual variability in psychosocial impairments. *Psychological Assessment, 34*(8), 777–790. https://doi.org/10.1037/pas0001139

De Los Reyes, A., & Epkins, C. C. (2023). Introduction to the special issue. A dozen years of demonstrating that informant discrepancies are more than measurement error: Toward guidelines for integrating data from multi-informant assessments of youth mental health. *Journal of Clinical Child and Adolescent Psychology, 52*(1), 1–18. https://doi.org/10.1080/15374416.2022.2158843

De Los Reyes, A., Epkins, C. C., Asmundson, G. J. G., Augenstein, T. M., Becker, K. D., Becker, S. P., Bonadio, F. T., Borelli, J. L., Boyd, R. C., Bradshaw, C. P., Burns, G. L., Casale, G., Causadias, J. M., Cha, C. B., Chorpita, B. F., Cohen, J. R., Comer, J. S., Crowell, S. E., Dirks, M. A., et al. (2023b). Editorial statement about *JCCAP*'s 2023 special issue on informant discrepancies in youth mental health assessments: Observations, guidelines, and future directions grounded in 60 years of research. *Journal of Clinical Child and Adolescent Psychology, 52*(1), 147–158. https://doi.org/10.1080/15374416.2022.2158842

De Los Reyes, A., Talbott, E., Power, T., Michel, J., Cook, C. R., Racz, S. J., & Fitzpatrick, O. (2022a). The Needs-to-Goals Gap: How informant discrepancies in youth mental health assessments impact service delivery. *Clinical Psychology Review, 92*, Article 102114. https://doi.org/10.1016/j.cpr.2021.102114

De Los Reyes, A., Tyrell, F. A., Watts, A. L., & Asmundson, G. J. G. (2022b). Conceptual, methodological, and measurement factors that disqualify use of measurement invariance techniques to detect informant discrepancies in youth mental health assessments. *Frontiers in Psychology, 13*, Article 931296. https://doi.org/10.3389/fpsyg.2022.931296

De Los Reyes, A., Wang, M., Lerner, M. D., Makol, B. A., Fitzpatrick, O., & Weisz, J. R. (2023a). The Operations Triad Model and youth mental health assessments: Catalyzing a paradigm shift in measurement validation. *Journal of Clinical Child and Adolescent Psychology, 52*(1), 19–54. https://doi.org/10.1080/15374416.2022.2111684

Dhillon, S., Bagby, R. M., Kushner, S. C., & Burchett, D. (2017). The impact of underreporting and overreporting on the validity of the personality inventory for DSM-5 (PID-5): A simulation analog design investigation. *Psychological Assessment, 29*(4), 473–478. https://doi.org/10.1037/pas0000359

Etkin, R. G., Lebowitz, E. R., & Silverman, W. K. (2021). Using evaluative criteria to review youth anxiety measures, part II: Parent-report. *Journal of Clinical Child and Adolescent Psychology, 50*(2), 155–176. https://doi.org/10.1080/15374416.2021.1878898

Eyberg, S. M., & Funderburk, B. (2011). *Parent-child interaction therapy protocol*. PCIT International.

Fadus, M. C., Ginsburg, K. R., Sobowale, K., Halliday-Boykins, C. A., Bryant, B. E., Gray, K. M., & Squeglia, L. M. (2020). Unconscious bias and the diagnosis of disruptive behavior disorders and ADHD in African American and Hispanic youth. *Academic Psychiatry, 44*(1), 95–102. https://doi.org/10.1007/s40596-019-01127-6

Garb, H. N. (2003). Incremental validity and the assessment of psychopathology in adults. *Psychological Assessment, 15*(4), 508–520. https://doi.org/10.1037/1040-3590.15.4.508

Gardner, T. W., Dishion, T. J., & Connell, A. M. (2008). Adolescent self-regulation as resilience: Resistance to antisocial behavior within the deviant peer context. *Journal of Abnormal Child Psychology, 36*(2), 273–284. https://doi.org/10.1007/s10802-007-9176-6

Goodman, S. H., Simon, H. F. M., Shamblaw, A. L., & Kim, C. Y. (2020). Parenting as a mediator of associations between depression in mothers and children's functioning: A systematic review and meta-analysis. *Clinical Child and Family Psychology Review, 23*(4), 427–460. https://doi.org/10.1007/s10567-020-00322-4

Greene, A. L., Eaton, N. R., Forbes, M. K., Fried, E. I., Watts, A. L., Kotov, R., & Krueger, R. F. (2022). Model fit is a fallible indicator of model quality in quantitative psychopathology research: A reply to Bader and Moshagen. *Journal of Psychopathology and Clinical Science, 131*(6), 696–703. https://doi.org/10.1037/abn0000770

Hunsley, J., & Mash, E. J. (2007). Evidence-based assessment. *Annual Review of Clinical Psychology, 3*, 29–51. https://doi.org/10.1146/annurev.clinpsy.3.022806.091419

Hurd, N. M., & Young, A. S. (2023). Introduction to the special issue: Advancing racial justice in clinical child and adolescent psychology. *Journal of Clinical Child and Adolescent Psychology, 52*(3), 311–327. https://doi.org/10.1080/15374416.2023.2202255

Jouriles, E. N., & Thompson, S. M. (1993). Effects of mood on mothers' evaluations of children's behavior. *Journal of Family Psychology, 6*(3), 300–307. https://doi.org/10.1037/0893-3200.6.3.300

Kang, S., & Harvey, E. A. (2020). Racial differences between black parents' and white teachers' perceptions of attention-deficit/hyperactivity disorder behavior. *Journal of Abnormal Child Psychology, 48*(5), 661–672. https://doi.org/10.1007/s10802-019-00600-y

Kline, R. B. (2016). *Principles and practice of structural equation modeling* (4th ed.). Guilford.

Lau, A. S., Garland, A. F., Yeh, M., Mccabe, K. M., Wood, P. A., & Hough, R. L. (2004). Race/ethnicity and inter-informant agreement in assessing adolescent psychopathology. *Journal of Emotional and Behavioral Disorders, 12*(3), 145–156. https://doi.org/10.1177/10634266040120030201

Lewis, C. C., Boyd, M., Puspitasari, A., Navarro, E., Howard, J., Kassab, H., ... & Kroenke, K. (2019). Implementing measurement-based care in behavioral health: A review. *JAMA Psychiatry, 76*(3), 324–335. https://doi.org/10.1001/jamapsychiatry.2018.3329

Lieberman, A. F., Ghosh Ippen, C., & Van Horn, P. J. (2015). *Don't hit my mommy: A manual for child-parent psychotherapy with young witnesses of family violence* (2nd ed.). Zero to Three.

Lindhiem, O., Vaughn-Coaxum, R. A., Higa, J., Harris, J. L., Kolko, D. J., & Pilkonis, P. A. (2020). Development and validation of the parenting skill use diary (PSUD) in a nationally representative sample. *Journal of Clinical Child and Adolescent Psychology, 50*(3), 400–410. https://doi.org/10.1080/15374416.2020.1716366

Luthar, S. S., Cicchetti, D., & Becker, B. (2000). The construct of resilience: A critical evaluation and guidelines for future work. *Child Development, 71*(3), 543–562. https://doi.org/10.1111/1467-8624.00164

Madsen, K. B., Rask, C. U., Olsen, J., Niclasen, J., & Obel, C. (2020). Depression-related distortions in maternal reports of child behaviour problems. *European Child and Adolescent Psychiatry, 29*(3), 275–285. https://doi.org/10.1007/s00787-019-01351-3

Marsh, J. K., Zeveney, A. S., & De Los Reyes, A. (2020). Informant discrepancies in judgments about change during mental health treatments. *Clinical Psychological Science, 8*(2), 318–332. https://doi.org/10.1177/2167702619894905

McLeod, B. D., Jensen-Doss, A., Lyon, A. R., Douglas, S., & Beidas, R. S. (2022). To utility and beyond! Specifying and advancing the utility of measurement-based care for youth. *Journal of Clinical Child and Adolescent Psychology, 51*(4), 375–388. https://doi.org/10.1080/15374416.2022.2042698

Millsap, E. (2011). *Statistical methods for studying measurement invariance*. Taylor and Francis.

Nunnally, J. C., & Bernstein, I. H. (1994). *Psychometric theory* (3rd ed.). McGraw-Hill.

Owens, E. B., & Hinshaw, S. P. (2016). Childhood conduct problems and young adult outcomes among women with childhood attention-deficit/hyperactivity disorder (ADHD). *Journal of Abnormal Psychology, 125*(2), 220–232. https://doi.org/10.1037/abn0000084

Price, M. A., Weisz, J. R., McKetta, S., Hollinsaid, N. L., Lattanner, M. R., Reid, A. E., & Hatzenbuehler, M. L. (2022). Meta-analysis: Are psychotherapies less effective for black youth in communities with higher levels of anti-black racism? *Journal of the American Academy of Child and Adolescent Psychiatry, 61*(6), 754–763. https://doi.org/10.1016/j.jaac.2021.07.808

Revelle, W. (2024). The seductive beauty of latent variable models: Or why I don't believe in the Easter bunny. *Personality and Individual Differences, 221*, 112552. https://doi.org/10.1016/j.paid.2024.112552

Richters, J. E. (1992). Depressed mothers as informants about their children: A critical review of the evidence for distortion. *Psychological Bulletin, 112*(3), 485–499. https://doi.org/10.1037/0033-2909.112.3.485

Rodriguez, C. M., Wittig, S. M. O., & Christl, M.-E. (2019). Psychometric evaluation of a brief assessment of parents' disciplinary alternatives. *Journal of Child and Family Studies, 28*(6), 1490–1501. https://doi.org/10.1007/s10826-019-01387-8

Scott, J. C., McDermott, E. R., Harris, A. N., Johnson, K. G., Pinderhughes, E. E., & Spencer, M. B. (2021). Looking through a kaleidoscope: The phenomenological ethnic-racial socialization conceptual model and its application to US black and Latino youth and families. *Journal of Social Issues, 77*(4), 1327–1350. https://doi.org/10.1111/josi.12480

Sprich, S. E., Safren, S. A., Finkelstein, D., Remmert, J. E., & Hammerness, P. (2016). A randomized controlled trial of cognitive behavioral therapy for ADHD in medication-treated adolescents. *Journal of Child Psychology and Psychiatry, 57*(11), 1218–1226. https://doi.org/10.1016/j.cbpra.2015.01.001

Tabachnick, B. G., & Fidell, L. S. (2013). *Using multivariate statistics* (6th ed.). Pearson.

Talbott, E., De Los Reyes, A., Kearns, D. M., Mancilla-Martinez, J., Cook, C. R., & Wang, M. (2023). Evidence-based assessment in special education research: Advancing the use of evidence in assessment tools and empirical processes. *Exceptional Children, 89*(4), 467–487. https://doi.org/10.1177/00144029231171092

Watts, A. L., Makol, B. A., Palumbo, I. M., De Los Reyes, A., Olino, T. M., Latzman, R. D., DeYoung, C. G., Wood, P. K., & Sher, K. J. (2022). How robust is the p-factor? Using multitrait-multimethod modeling to inform the meaning of general factors of psychopathology in youth. *Clinical Psychological Science, 10*(4), 640–661. https://doi.org/10.1177/21677026211055170

West, A. E., Conn, B. M., Preston, E. G., & Dews, A. A. (2023). Dismantling structural racism in child and adolescent psychology: A call to action to transform healthcare, education, child welfare, and the psychology workforce to effectively promote BIPOC youth health and development. *Journal of Clinical Child and Adolescent Psychology, 52*(3), 427–446. https://doi.org/10.1080/15374416.2023.2202253

Youngstrom, E. A., Izard, C., & Ackerman, B. (1999). Dysphoria-related bias in maternal ratings of children. *Journal of Consulting and Clinical Psychology, 67*(6), 905–916. https://doi.org/10.1037/0022-006X.67.6.905

Index

B. A. Makol et al., *Youth Development in Context*, Springer Series on Child and Family Studies, https://doi.org/10.1007/978-3-031-80549-3